# PROSPECTIVE PAYMENT

## Managing for Operational Effectiveness

**Howard L. Smith, Ph.D.**
Associate Professor, Department of Health Administration
Medical College of Virginia

**Myron D. Fottler, Ph.D.**
Professor of Management and Director of the Ph.D. Program
in Administration-Health Services
University of Alabama at Birmingham

AN ASPEN PUBLICATION®
Aspen Systems Corporation

1985

Rockville, Maryland
Royal Tunbridge Wells

Library of Congress Cataloging in Publication Data

Smith, Howard L.
Prospective payment.

"An Aspen publication."
Includes bibliographies and index.
1. Hospitals—Prospective payment. 2. Hospitals—Rates. 3. Hospitals—
Planning. I. Fottler, Myron D. II. Title.
RA971.3.S57     1985     362.1'1'0681     85-1294
ISBN: 0-87189-097-6

Editorial Services: Ruth Bloom

Library of Congress Catalog Card Number: 85-1294
ISBN: 0-87189-097-6

Printed in the United States of America

1  2  3  4  5

# Table of Contents

# Preface

*Prospective Payment: Managing for Operational Effectiveness* was written as a response to significant changes in hospital reimbursement—the development of diagnosis-related groups (DRGs) and the implementation of prospective payment. Because few hospital executives have planned for such a revolution in the manner by which hospitals are paid for their services, they need guidelines that pragmatically address strategy formulation and tactical planning. They also need a book that they can distribute to trustees, who need to understand the strategic implications of DRG-based reimbursement for their hospitals, and to key department heads and supervisors, who need to know what specific actions they can take in response to DRGs.

Since other major third party payers are following the lead of Medicare and adopting prospective payment systems, it is clear that a revolutionary era has been ushered in for hospitals. Management strategy must be revised to address the changes. While hospital executives must implement specific operating changes to meet the challenges of prospective payment, they should be concerned first with their strategic plans. Unless those plans are of sufficient vision, their hospitals are unlikely to remain financially solvent and healthy in the prospective payment environment.

*Prospective Payment* provides a managerial perspective on the various strategic and tactical factors that must be modified under prospective payment. It is a convenient starting point from which hospitals can be managed in an era of cost control.

Finally, this book can serve as an integrative text in graduate and undergraduate health administration courses, such as health care financing, strategic planning, and overview courses. It has been written with these major courses in mind.

# Acknowledgments

Howard L. Smith extends his appreciation to the Anderson Schools of Management at the University of New Mexico and the Department of Health Administration at the Medical College of Virginia for their support of his research and teaching related to health services administration.

Lynne Yaple at QA Typing deserves mention for her effort to produce a coherent product from indecipherable writing.

Finally, special thanks go to his family and friends for pardoning transgressions during the process of writing this book.

Myron D. Fottler thanks several individuals at the University of Alabama in Birmingham (UAB) who made significant contributions to this book. Jeffrey Albright, an M.B.A. candidate in the Graduate School of Management, made a major contribution to the final outcome through his thorough and detailed library research and summaries of the literature concerning prospective payment and DRGs. Joyce Lanning, a Ph.D. candidate in Administration-Health Services, lent the author her voluminous materials on the topic; these were particularly helpful for Chapters 2 and 11.

Several secretaries at UAB typed portions of the manuscript, including Pat Washington and Judy Mitchell of the School of Business and Val Ostrosky and Selina Todd of the School of Community and Allied Health. Both Dean Gene Newport of the School of Business and Dean Keith Blayney of the School of Community and Allied Health at UAB deserve recognition for their continued support of the Ph.D. program in general and this research and publication in particular.

In addition, many thanks to Nena Sanders, a faculty member of the School of Nursing at UAB, for providing materials relevant to Chapter 12 as well as valuable comments on the first draft of that chapter.

Finally, Dr. Fottler would like to acknowledge a debt of gratitude to his wife, Carol.

# Chapter 1

# The Path to Prospective Payment Systems

These days one can hardly read a health care journal without being confronted with phrases such as prospective payment system (PPS) and diagnosis-related groups (DRGs). The Tax Equity and Fiscal Responsibility Act of 1982 (P.L. 97–248) and the Social Security Amendments of 1983 (P.L. 98–21) mandated that, beginning in October 1983, hospitals be reimbursed for the costs of care provided to Medicare patients at a flat illness-specific rate that is established prospectively.

Under the previous retrospective reimbursement system, hospitals were reimbursed *after* they rendered services. This system encouraged hospitals to utilize services and raise costs because reimbursement was reasonably assured for every service. The new prospective payment system, under which hospitals are paid an amount fixed *in advance,* is an effort to encourage efficiency and contain hospital costs.

The flat amount paid for the care of each Medicare patient is determined by the patient's diagnosis, which must fit into one of 467 DRGs. Researchers developed these DRGs on the basis of the factors that contribute significantly to hospital resource consumption (e.g., complications, age, and any surgical procedures performed). Each DRG has a predetermined dollar "price," calculated as the average cost per case in that DRG category. With some modifications, these are the amounts that the federal government now pays hospitals for patient care, even if the actual costs are higher or lower.

## THE COST PROBLEM

The health care field has witnessed steadily rising costs over the last several decades. The inflationary effect of these increasing costs has received considerable attention. Yet, despite the efforts of hospital administrators, medical staff,

1

nonmedical staff, and consumers to contain them, health care costs continue to increase at a rate greater than the rate of general inflation; an effective solution has yet to be developed and implemented. The immediate result of this failure to control hospital costs is the development of new public policies, such as PPSs. Many third party insurers are also adopting prospective payment as a method of controlling health care costs.

In some cases, hospitals themselves have not been directly responsible for the increased cost levels. They have experienced a climate of inflationary costs over which they have no control. For example, the proliferation of sophisticated medical technologies, the limited consumer cost caring, the construction of unneeded hospital beds, and the development of nonreimbursable programs or services have all contributed to runaway hospital costs. In reality, no single institution is responsible for the predicament in which today's hospitals find themselves. Government agencies, third party reimbursers, the public, health care professionals, and health care organizations have all contributed to excessive hospital costs. In essence, there has been no incentive to contain costs.

Hospital executives must now determine how best to manage their facilities in view of the public concern over health care costs. Essentially, they must study the present environment, consider possible future changes, and develop both tactical and strategic interventions that will help ensure survival and success. Virtually every hospital executive must plan for the changes resulting from prospective payment. The other concerns that have required the attention of hospital executives in the past may have to be set aside temporarily while the effects of prospective payment are analyzed.

Although daily problems, such as capital financing, staff productivity, quality of care, promotion of services, malpractice litigation, nursing staff shortages, unions, bad debts, and charitable care, will continue to plague hospitals, the economic environment for hospitals has changed dramatically. So, too, must the managerial reactions to that environment change. Eventually, plans for management under a PPS must be integrated into daily decision making, since such a system will alter significantly the strategic management of hospitals. This profound change in reimbursement may motivate hospitals to gain control over the cost of services provided. Furthermore, the manipulation of hospital reimbursement may make it possible to implement internal changes that would never have been made under traditional payment mechanisms.

## EARLIER ATTEMPTS TO CONTROL HEALTH CARE COSTS

Prospective payment systems have been preceded by a long history of public policy measures aimed at controlling health care costs. Despite the ineffectiveness of these measures in actually controlling costs, they have had an indelible impact on hospitals. Significant policy and operational modifications have been introduced and institutionalized in hospitals as a result of these policies. It is inevitable that other modifications will occur with any change in reimbursement policies.

In the last two decades, four major health policies have been implemented in an effort to control health care costs: (1) health planning (i.e., comprehensive health planning and health systems agencies); (2) professional standards review organizations (PSROs); (3) health maintenance organizations (HMOs); and (4) cost sharing by third party payers. Except perhaps for HMOs, hospital executives have been encouraged to incorporate these policies into the plans and daily operations of their hospitals. Yet, the success of these policies has been limited in controlling costs, since the basic incentive structure in hospitals was not significantly altered.

## Health Planning

Because the presence of unneeded hospital beds has been associated with higher health care costs in many communities, comprehensive health planning was instituted to reduce duplication of services and facilities by proposing local plans for the construction or expansion of health care facilities and for the purchase of major equipment. The purpose of planning was to encourage more efficient use of existing facilities and equipment in hospitals (and other health care facilities), which ultimately would reduce health care costs.

Hospital executives soon discovered that health planning presented a unique set of constraints. No longer could they build new facilities or purchase major equipment whenever they deemed it necessary. Now an external agency that was often hostile to further expansion of hospital plant and equipment had to approve these strategic decisions. Furthermore, health planning policy failed to contain costs because it overlooked a major determinant of rising costs—the internal operation of hospitals.

In the end, health planning has come to serve little more than a review function. It has been criticized not only for failing to contain costs, but also for delaying construction, which ultimately allowed costs to increase. Many hospitals watched construction costs multiply while health planning agencies deliberated on various certificate-of-need proposals. Today, many of these process problems have been resolved. Nonetheless, hospital executives have learned that it is necessary to undertake a deliberate analysis of the implications of any proposed cost containment policy, or their hospitals may find themselves in a disadvantageous position from which it is difficult to recover. Hospitals that planned for construction while the health planning policy was being formulated, for example, found that their timely reaction to health planning allowed them to improve their financial position over time; their resources were not expended in lengthy certificate-of-need reviews, and financing could be obtained at reasonable rates.

## Professional Standards Review Organizations

In conjunction with the health planning policies, PSROs were implemented, ostensibly to control the quality of medical services. There are several interpretations of the implied and real goals of PSROs. It is often suggested that PSROs were designed to identify those physicians who contributed to rising costs by admitting patients to the hospital unnecessarily, by requiring longer than necessary lengths of stay, or by performing inappropriate or unneeded procedures. Hospitals responded to the goals of PSROs by forming or expanding utilization review committees and medical audit committees. These committees attempted to control unnecessary use internally.

Like health planning agencies, PSROs have been hampered by a confusing organizational structure, disjointed and incremental funding, and the lack of a clear mission or purpose. They failed to contain costs because of the problems in defining appropriate versus unnecessary care. It is possible that more resources have been expended in identifying outliers than have been saved in correcting deficiencies. Furthermore, PSROs have not contained costs on an institutionwide basis, since they have focused primarily on physicians, excluding nonmedical staff and consumers. Once again, hospital executives have learned a valuable lesson about public policy attempts at cost control—in order to have maximum effectiveness within hospitals, the policy must provide incentives for cost containment among consumers, as well as among all hospital staff members.

## Health Maintenance Organizations

Prepaid health plans or HMOs have been moderately successful in reducing costs through disease prevention and shorter average lengths of hospitalization. HMOs have failed to establish themselves on a pervasive basis across the United States, however, despite assistance from the federal government for planning and initial operational funding.

Hospitals are involved in HMOs as providers of inpatient care, but hospitals usually are either associated with a single HMO or the HMO patients compete with other patients who are reimbursed through several mechanisms. As a result, the general effectiveness of HMOs as a method of controlling costs is rather limited. Advocates of HMOs continue to support the expansion of the prepaid concept, however. It remains to be seen whether the government will develop further incentives in the future to attract hospitals to HMO care. For the moment, most hospitals are concentrating on acute episodic care, because they are not associated with a prepaid group.

Even though the HMO has shown promise as a method for controlling costs, it has not been widely accepted by health care consumers, who are attuned to solo practitioners and family physicians. They may be reluctant to modify their purchase of health care services if these services deviate from perceived normal patterns of care, even when intrahospital changes benefit consumers by controlling costs.

## Cost Sharing

Public and private third party insurers have tried to contain costs through deductibles and co-payment. This cost sharing has been successful in containing consumer demand, but the regressive nature of the deductibles and co-payments on the indigent and marginally poor have prevented further expansion of the concept in the health care field. The main principle of importance to hospital executives is the role of economic incentives. Cost sharing has proved to be more effective than other policy interventions in controlling costs. Its success is based on the economic incentive for consumers, which helps prevent them from over-utilizing services. The same principle can be applied to hospitals; staff members can participate in incentive programs that are advantageous (in terms of economic or noneconomic rewards) to both individual and hospital.

## REIMBURSEMENT POLICIES

There is a long history of experimentation with hospital reimbursement for health care by the federal and state governments. Collectively, however, this experience has produced more confusion than understanding in regard to the ideal model for hospital reimbursement. Although there are several alternate payment mechanisms, two reimbursement systems are prevalent—retrospective payment and prospective payment.

## Retrospective Reimbursement

Under a retrospective payment system, hospitals are reimbursed for services on a cost basis; after services have been provided, hospitals are reimbursed for the costs generated in the provision of those services. There is very little incentive, if any, to control the level of expenditures for hospital services under this system because hospitals are not penalized if costs increase. The hospital can simply pass any increases in the costs that it incurs to the third party payers. If the cost of internal resources (e.g., labor) rises, reimbursable costs increase. If the cost of external resources (e.g., utilities, supplies, equipment) rises, these costs can also be submitted by the hospital for reimbursement. As a result of this third party reimbursement, costs increased uncontrollably whenever a new technology appeared or the cost of input factors increased. Attempts to harness the factors from which hospital costs are derived (e.g., by establishing standard fee scales and negotiated rates) were not comprehensive and generally of insufficient magnitude to make hospitals conscientious about cost control. Instead, hospitals resorted to elaborate tactics by which they shifted costs—usually to private pay patients or full paying insurance carriers—to maintain solvency.

The practical significance of retrospective payments for hospital executives is often overlooked. The system's effect is simple yet extraordinarily powerful, however. A retrospective payment system fails to motivate sound management practices. Without an incentive to control costs, hospital executives need not worry about establishing planning, decision-making, control, and incentive systems within their organizations. They have a greater opportunity to function merely as caretakers of a complex organization.

## Prospective Reimbursement

In a prospective reimbursement system, hospitals are cognizant of the amount that they will receive in funding for a given set of services before they actually provide the services. Prospective reimbursement encourages hospitals to contain costs—if the payment rate is set near the level of costs. Since all hospitals (whether nonprofit or for-profit) must have at least an accounting rate of return on their investment in order to maintain capital assets, the reimbursing agent can encourage cost control by establishing a reimbursement rate that is slightly above real costs.

Studies of prospective reimbursement for hospitals in several states have suggested that these payment systems do indeed help to contain costs.[1,2] The results also indicate, however, that the progress in cost containment is very slow and that it may take perhaps several years to meaningfully slow the increase in hospital expenditures. Furthermore, although prospective payment is promising as a mechanism for controlling costs, confusing and arbitrary processes may be followed in determining the rate level.

## Evolution of Hospital Reimbursement in the United States

The traditional payment system is retrospective and per diem as shown in Cell 1 of Figure 1–1. The present Medicare reimbursement system is best represented by Cell 4, which is a prospective payment system calculated per diagnosis (not per diem). If the new system had been based on prospective payment per diem (Cell 2), the change would have been less significant; many private insurance and Medicaid programs are already under such a per diem prospective payment system and have been for several years. That approach is presently being discarded, however, because it has been found to reduce necessary utilization. Thus, the change is not only a shift from retrospective to prospective reimbursement, but also a shift from per diem to per diagnosis reimbursement.

**Figure 1–1** Evolution of Hospital Reimbursement Systems

| | Timing of Payment | |
|---|---|---|
| Unit of Payment | Retrospective | Prospective |
| Per diem | 1 | 2 |
| Per diagnosis | 3 | 4 |

The failure of hospital executives to devise and implement sound management principles under a system of retrospective reimbursement is a legacy that will seriously affect hospitals when a prospective payment system is implemented. Many hospitals will discover that they are incapable of modifying their management philosophies or of orchestrating their resources in meeting the challenges presented by the new system. It is not too late to revise the methods of managing, however, since prospective payment (for Medicare) is to be phased in over a three-year period. Yet, every delay raises a barrier to an operationally feasible system that meets the demands of prospective reimbursement.

The management weaknesses wrought by retrospective reimbursement are most evident in planning, control, and staff incentives. Practically speaking, hospital executives must attend to these areas at least if they expect to fare well under a prospective payment system. An entirely new, more rigorous philosophy of management must be introduced so that hospitals are managed with operationally measurable and attainable standards of efficiency and effectiveness. This revolution will require several basic changes.

Under a prospective payment system, hospitals must have planning systems solidly in place in order to identify their goals—particularly clinical service areas. Under retrospective payment systems, hospitals could rely on ad hoc decision making and planning because there was little pressure to ensure financial solvency; financial goals were easily attainable under conditions of full (or nearly full) cost reimbursement. Therefore, budgeting was a relatively meaningless activity, and deviations from planned goals aroused little concern. Staff had little incentive for improving the hospital's performance, because they were not held accountable for deviations from anticipated performance.

Hospital executives must recognize that reimbursement based on DRGs, or a variation of it, will characterize future hospital payments. DRGs can influence virtually every aspect of hospital service because they change the incentive system under which hospitals operate. If hospital executives are alert to this trend and undertake sufficient prior preparation, DRG-based reimbursement should have no substantial impact on the quality and harmony of the hospital environment. There may be changes, even major changes, in the manner in which tasks are completed or in standard operating procedures, but the certainty of the hospital environment need not be severely jeopardized.

Hospital executives must formulate strategic and tactical plans, and must implement them carefully. Under the DRG system, hospitals will have to fine-tune their operations if they expect to survive financially. Hospital executives are responsible not only for fine-tuning operations, but also for buffering medical and non-medical staff against the confusion that may accompany the implementation of the DRG system. Therefore, hospital executives require a practical perspective on DRG-based reimbursement. They need more than just a philosophy to negotiate the hazards and constraints presented by DRGs; they need a complete vision—a model—of a hospital's movement from retrospective to prospective reimbursement. This model must be comprehensive and easily translated into specific operational actions.

## A PRACTICAL MANAGEMENT MODEL FOR DRG-BASED REIMBURSEMENT

Figure 1–2 shows the four major components of the management model of DRG-based reimbursement: (1) external environmental changes leading to prospective payment, (2) strategic factors, (3) tactical factors, and (4) outcomes of effectively managing the constraints of prospective payment.

### Environmental Changes

The environmental shift from retrospective to prospective reimbursement is complex; it requires philosophical changes in hospital executives, as well as practical managerial changes. It is easy to dismiss the philosophical change as academic or irrelevant, but the failure of hospitals in the past to emphasize cost containment in their management philosophy has resulted in the current implementation of major regulatory/reimbursement interventions.

The internal management of a hospital is determined by the environment (or context) in which it exists. This is the popular and empirically substantiated view of the contingency approach to management. Both strategic and operating variables must be managed in response to the pressures presented by the external environment. The better the match between the external environment and internal operations, the higher the level of performance attained by the hospital. This relationship has been tested in many organizations with considerable success.

Even though prospective payment systems may vary from state to state, they are very much alike in their ultimate impact on hospitals. The imposition of these reimbursement systems influences the management strategies within hospitals.

**Figure 1-2** Management Model for DRG-Based Reimbursement

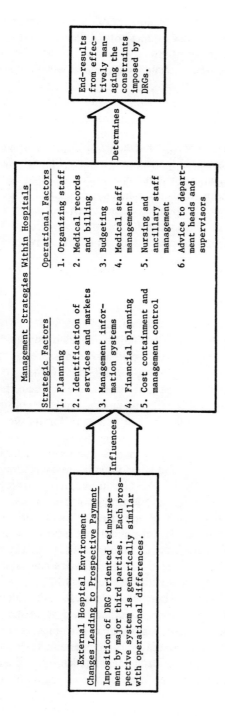

The degree of influence and the match between the hospital and its reimbursement environment are contingent, of course, on the sensitivity of the management staff to the external pressures. If hospital executives are cognizant of these pressures, they are likely to modify the strategic and tactical elements of hospital services.

## Strategic Factors

Hospital executives must address at least five strategic management factors in their response to prospective payment: (1) the planning system, (2) identification of services and markets, (3) management information systems, (4) financial planning, and (5) cost containment programs with management control. The exact number of strategic factors with which hospital executives must deal is determined by the hospital and the history of its management. If properly developed, however, these five strategic variables will give a hospital the opportunity to thrive under the constraints imposed by prospective payments.

### Planning

The implementation of DRG-based reimbursement can be viewed as an opportunity for strengthening hospital planning. Hospital executives must plan future responses to prospective reimbursement rather than wait for pressures to force a reaction; otherwise, the executives are allowing the situation to manage them instead of vice versa. It may be necessary to overcome a high degree of inertia, however, since few hospital executives find planning a glamorous responsibility. Even so, the planning function has always been a key factor in successful organizations.

Hospital executives must address both short-term and long-term plans. First, it must be determined how to get organized and who to involve in the planning and decision-making processes surrounding DRGs. Generally, more medical and nonmedical staff members, who can provide a wider array of expertise, are needed for planning under prospective payment than are needed under retrospective payment. Attention should then shift to the formation of a short-term survival plan. This plan may involve, for example, identification of DRGs that are deviant (i.e., that are producing excessive costs) and define strategies and tactics for improving the management of those DRGs within the hospital.

Long-term planning can build on the short-term plans. Key considerations include maintaining staff interest in cost containment, selecting alternative strategies for containing costs in the future, analyzing resource investments to produce the best response to DRG-based reimbursement, revising operations schedules to speed up the attainment of cost-effective performance, and identifying the DRGs that apply to the mission of the hospital.

## Determination of Services and Markets

In their efforts to provide comprehensive care, hospitals have become very generalized. Some DRGs are more lucrative than others, however. Caseloads may not be sufficient to justify the continued provision of some services, or equipment may be too expensive to permit continuation of those services for which revenues do not cover costs. Thus, hospitals will be forced to be more selective when determining the DRGs for which they will provide care.

DRGs will also play an important role in hospital program development. Hospital executives must undertake a critical evaluation of the programs and services offered. Cost-effective services and programs will be maintained and allowed to expand, unprofitable services and programs that can be made profitable will require increased marketing, and those that cannot be made profitable will be discontinued. Some unprofitable services may be continued, however, if they help to reduce unit fixed costs. For example, a particular service may generate insufficient revenue to cover the total unit costs (fixed and variable) of providing the service, but the hospital may continue to offer the service if the alternative is a large number of empty beds that make no contribution to reducing fixed costs per patient day. The executives must also make decisions at this time involving charitable care and the capacity of the hospital to maintain its contribution in the face of declining reimbursement.

Under the new DRG-based reimbursement system, the cost of treating a patient with a particular diagnosis in a given hospital is not necessarily correlated with the amount that Medicare will pay for this treatment. Although they should theoretically be equal in a statistically "average" hospital, almost all hospitals will show costs that are greater or less than this average. Consequently, most DRGs will be "winners" or "losers" for a given hospital.

## Hospital Management Information Systems

It will be impossible to manage DRGs without necessary information. Hospital executives will have to define who, what, when, where, and how information needs will be fulfilled. The information system must be designed to emphasize decision variables and information relevant to those decisions, such as case mix, average length of stay, productivity, identification of DRG outliers, and identification of both medical and nonmedical staff members who are responsible for excessive costs.

## Financial Planning

Special attention must be focused on the financial area in planning, specifically on the changing income statement and balance sheets in hospitals. Hospital executives must identify those services or departments that produce surplus revenues that can be shared with other operating areas.

Financial planning under a DRG-based reimbursement system requires an increased emphasis on facility and equipment decisions. Hospital capital has been eroding under retrospective payment, and this trend will be exacerbated under prospective payment unless hospitals begin to plan very rigorously for their expenditures on new plant and equipment. Under Medicare, capital costs will be integrated with prospective payment in 1986. Thus, hospitals are forewarned that future capital needs will have to be met at least partially by retention of funds from current operations.

Although many scenarios are still possible in the financial area, it appears likely that patients may eventually be integrated into cost sharing with hospitals, especially since third party payers will have considerable control over the amount reimbursed and, in some cases, over rate increases. Patient cost sharing may be used to compensate for deficits. Furthermore, financial planning may reinforce the importance of minimizing bad debts so that hospitals may become even more cautious about admitting patients who have a questionable ability to pay.

### Management Control

The very essence of a DRG-based reimbursement system is the effort to control the level of health care expenditures by forcing hospitals to become more cost-effective and efficient. Fortunately, there is a growing interest among hospital executives in identifying practical methods for controlling costs. In addition, health services research has established a foundation of knowledge that can be very useful in developing specific management strategies to control costs under prospective payment.

## Tactical Factors

In responding to a DRG-based prospective payment system, hospital executives must carefully manage at least six tactical factors: (1) staff organization, (2) medical records and billing, (3) budgeting, (4) medical staff management, (5) nursing and ancillary staff management, and (6) departmental supervision. Each of these factors is a critical element in the daily management of a DRG-based system.

### Staff Organization

A variety of staff organizational formats can be implemented in the hospital to ensure that DRGs receive an optimum degree of attention. Some hospitals may establish a coordinator or designate a department or task force to manage the internal ramifications of DRGs. The success of a DRG management program hinges on the commitment given to the DRG coordinator (or department) by the top administrators and by the board of directors, however. Furthermore, the medical staff must participate in this group commitment. Once the level of commitment has been established and reinforced, it becomes a matter of integrating the DRG program into other planning and decision-making functions in the hospital.

## Medical Records and Billing

Because hospitals want to be reimbursed for the highest paying DRG for each case, hospital executives must manage several areas in medical records and billing departments. Medical records must be kept in a way that permits the final diagnosis to be identified for billing. It may be necessary to upgrade the in-service education of medical records and billing clerks to achieve this end. It may even be appropriate to establish a system of rewards for departmental supervisors and staff members to underscore the importance of correct diagnosis coding and billing.

## Budgeting

In the past, some hospitals have viewed budgeting as a superfluous activity. Although useful for guidance, budgets were never considered a really important aspect of operations. The outcome of this approach has been a rather senseless cycle in which budgets are formulated by the financial staff, reviewed by the administration and department heads, and virtually forgotten until the next round of budgeting. Departments have not been adequately rewarded for achieving their budgets or sufficiently penalized for failing to achieve them. As part of a rigorous internal planning process, however, budgeting must also be integrated into a system of control. The implementation of DRG-based reimbursement will motivate executives to identify where costs are excessive and to apply a system of incentives to bring these costs under control.

## Medical Staff Management

Many of the tactical factors that have been discussed are related to the performance of staff members and their ability to adjust to the new demands imposed by prospective reimbursement. Hospital executives must carefully manage both medical and nonmedical staff members. Physicians will probably be reluctant to modify their patterns of practice, even when the hospital encourages (or pressures) them to diagnose their patients' medical condition in the most severe DRG. This pressure comes naturally as part of the effort to ensure maximum reimbursement for the care of each patient. Physicians have been vocal about these pressures for ''DRG creep'' when a hospital's case mix severity increases suddenly for no demonstrable medical reason. Physicians may also find that their medical staff privileges have suddenly become very restricted unless they can substantiate their ability to make a financial contribution to the hospital. The pressures are economic, hence managerial. Hospital executives must be sensitive to physician attitudes about DRG management; they must keep the staff informed about their management plans for DRGs. Without the cooperation of the medical staff in the management of the DRG-based reimbursement system, the hospital's financial condition will deteriorate, and both the medical and the management staffs will be seeking another facility in which to practice.

*Ancillary Staff Management*

The nursing and ancillary staff occupy a position that is similar in many respects to that of physicians. Hospital executives generally have greater control over the ancillary staff than over the medical staff, and they must capitalize on this advantage. Operational methods of achieving this control include in-service education, ancillary staff participation in planning for cost containment, creation of incentive programs, and monitoring of ancillary staff productivity.

It is imperative that hospital executives develop at the department head and supervisory level the sort of leadership that encourages maximum response to the constraints of DRGs. Effective leadership and supervision under which staff members are led to high productivity and quality performance will no longer suffice; these goals must be achieved under the added demands of a prospective payment system. Hospitals will need executives who are prepared to help department heads and supervisors set new staff performance standards that are compatible with cost reduction. Especially critical will be the specification of measurable objectives for departments and for individuals.

## Outcomes

By being sensitive to the external environment that has led to prospective payment and by forming strategic and tactical plans to address the environmental shift, hospital executives should be able to progress toward improved hospital performance.

---

**NOTES**

1. Frank A. Sloan and Bruce Steinwald, "Effects of Regulation on Hospital Cost and Use," *Journal of Law and Economics* 23 (1980):81–109.

2. Craig Coelen and Daniel Sullivan, "An Analysis of the Effects of Prospective Reimbursement Programs on Hospital Expenditures," *Health Care Financing Review* 5(1981):1–40.

# Chapter 2

# Prospective Rate Setting Based on DRGs

Medicare was created to make medical care available to the elderly, but the achievement of the original legislative goal has been hampered by rising health care costs. In 1967, Medicare paid approximately $3.2 billion for hospital services; in 1983, Medicare expenditures were approximately $37 billion. Moreover, when the rate of inflation rose 5 percent in 1982, hospital costs rose 15.5 percent. Finally, the deductible for Medicare hospital insurance had risen from $40 in 1967 to $304 in 1983.[1]

With massive federal budget deficits and expectations that Medicare costs will reach $110 billion in 1987, both the Reagan Administration and Congress recognized the need for Medicare reform.[2]

Although interest in prospective reimbursement for health care costs began in 1972, there was no mandate to develop it until 1982, when the Tax Equity and Fiscal Responsibility Act (TEFRA) was enacted. The major hospital reimbursement changes in TEFRA were:

1. a limit on total inpatient costs per discharge, adjusted to reflect each hospital's case mix of patients
2. a limit on the annual rate of increase of total costs per discharge
3. a small incentive payment for hospitals that keep costs below both of these limits

These interim reimbursement reforms of TEFRA were accompanied by a provision that directed the secretary of Health and Human Services (HHS) to propose long-range Medicare reimbursement reforms with built-in incentives for hospital management efficiency. Thus, in December 1982, secretary of HHS Richard Schweiker proposed that the method by which hospitals are compensated for Medicare patient services be changed to a system based on diagnosis-related groups (DRGs). This proposal was adopted by Congress (P.L. 98-21) and signed into law on April 20, 1983 by President Reagan.

This action continued the movement, begun in 1982, away from retrospective, cost-based reimbursement as a basis for hospital payment by the Medicare program to a new prospective payment system. Unlike the TEFRA, the new prospective payment system based on DRGs sets a reimbursable amount for each DRG rather than establishing a case mix–adjusted cost-per-case limit for the hospital, severs the traditional relationship between revenues and costs, and puts the hospital fully "at risk" for differences between average costs within the DRGs and the DRG payment.

This is the initial step toward long-term financial stability in the Medicare program, because it allows hospitals to benefit financially (for the first time) from improvements in management. Prospective reimbursement creates financial incentives for hospitals to use their resources carefully in providing inpatient care. Reimbursement payments are now fixed at the beginning of the year, and costs must be kept within the limits of available resources. In addition, physician involvement in the management of patient services is essential, since the hospital is "at risk" for the patient mix, the use of services, and the length of stay within each DRG.

## THE CASE MIX CONCEPT

The term *case mix* is used to describe the numbers and types of patients treated in a hospital. When the case mix concept was first developed, researchers concentrated on the institution-related variables, such as average length of stay, medical school affiliation, bed size, and provision of particular clinical services. Currently, researchers define case mix in terms of patient-related variables, such as diagnosis, personal characteristics (e.g., age), and acuity. Patients who are similar, as defined by the assignment criteria, are grouped into the same categories.[3]

Studies conducted throughout the 1970s indicated that significant cost variations among hospitals could be explained by differences in case mix.[4] In an early study of 177 British hospitals, Feldstein found that patient case mix could account for 25 percent of the variation in per case costs.[5] Goodisman and Trompeter, in a more recent study, used charge per case as the dependent variable and found case mix accounted for 58 percent of interhospital variation.[6] The relationship between hospital costs and case mix becomes intuitively evident when the medical needs of patients are described in terms of complexity (i.e., the types of services provided) and intensity (i.e., the numbers of services provided). Case mix measures incorporate both, since hospital costs are correlated with the number and complexity of services needed to treat each patient.[7]

There is a trade-off involved in all attempts to fit patients into case mix groups. If all patient characteristics are used, the resulting classifications will be overly numerous, statistically insignificant, and administratively burdensome. On the other hand, when categories are combined, some legitimate differences are lost. The extent to which patients can be combined into meaningful groups depends on their homogeneity.

Satisfactory case mix classifications should be medically, economically, and administratively homogeneous.[8] Medical homogeneity involves the extent to which patients within categories have similar clinical conditions or treatment regimens; patients assigned to the same group should have similar treatments and prognoses. Economic homogeneity requires groups of patients to be reasonably similar in terms of their resource consumption. This is necessary for equality in establishing prospective payment rates based on case mix.[9] In fact, the extent to which payment based on a case mix measure is appropriate is largely dependent on the extent to which patient classifications are economically homogeneous.[10] Patient classification categories that are both economically and medically homogeneous tend to be most effective because they provide a common language for hospital financial managers and the medical staff.[11] Finally, a satisfactory patient classification system must be easily administered rather than burdensome to the user.

## EVOLUTION OF DRGs

DRGs were developed primarily at Yale–New Haven Hospital by Robert Fetter and John Thompson, who began their research in 1970 with the objective of improving the utilization review process. The original DRGs were based on the broad groupings of the *International Classification of Diseases–Eighth Revision–Clinical Modification* (ICD–8–CM). Using a large data base of hospital records from New Jersey, Connecticut, and South Carolina, clinicians grouped diagnoses in accordance with three principles. Categories were established (1) to group diagnoses consistent in their anatomical, physiological classification (i.e., the manner in which they are clinically managed); (2) to be large enough to represent statistically meaningful patient populations; and (3) to cover the range of ICD–8–CM categories without overlap. The result was a list of 83 major diagnostic categories.

An interactive computerized algorithm was then used to split the major diagnostic categories into groups that contained more than 100 cases. On completion of this process, it was decided that additional groups must be even further subdivided in order to reduce the variance in length of hospital stay within groups. Therefore, secondary diagnoses, primary surgical procedure, age, and absence or presence of a particular service were incorporated into the grouping process, resulting in a total of 383 DRGs.[12]

A second generation of DRGs was developed in 1981 in response to a new disease-coding scheme, the *International Classification of Diseases–Ninth Revision–Clinical Modification* (ICD–9–CM). The new DRGs were based on a nationwide sample of 400,000 medical records of patients discharged during the first half of 1979. These records were selected from 332 of 2,100 hospitals participating in the Commission on Professional and Hospital Activities data service. A panel of physicians divided all ICD–9–CM diagnosis codes into 23 major diagnostic categories based on the body system affected (e.g., digestive, respiratory). The major diagnostic categories were then subdivided according to the performance of a surgical procedure, the principal diagnosis, the presence of a complicating condition, patient age, sex, and discharge status. This resulted in 467 DRGs.[13] The presence or absence of an operating room procedure is the first major subdivision within most major diagnostic categories because of the high cost and staff requirements associated with such procedures (Figure 2–1). The second partitioning of patients is predicated on the presence or absence of a complication (i.e., a secondary condition that arises during hospitalization) or comorbidity (i.e., a condition that coexisted at admission with a specific principal diagnosis) that is expected to increase the length of stay by at least one day for about 75 percent of the patients.[14]

## SPECIFICS OF THE LEGISLATION

The Social Security Amendments of 1983 (Title VI), which legislated a prospective system for Medicare hospital payments, apply to all short-term acute care hospitals. These hospitals have been operating under a prospective payment system since the beginning of their first Medicare reporting year that began on or after October 1, 1983. Pediatric, long-term care (average length of stay greater than 25 days), psychiatric, and rehabilitation hospitals are exempt. Certain "distinct part" psychiatric and rehabilitation units of general hospitals may also be exempted by request if the secretary of HHS approves the request. Hospitals designated as "sole community providers" and rural hospitals with fewer than 50 beds may also receive exemptions. Hospitals are reimbursed for outpatient services and those services provided by exempted distinct units on a retrospective cost basis.

### DRG Payment Determination

The basis of hospital reimbursement under the prospective payment system is the discharge diagnosis of the particular patient. The payment rate for each DRG is

**Figure 2-1** Classification Scheme for Major Diagnostic Category 4, Diseases and Disorders of the Respiratory System (DRGs 75–86)

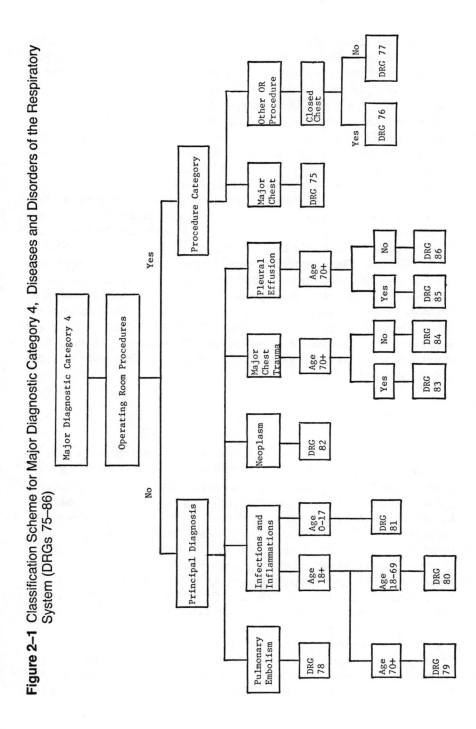

established on the basis of three sources of data: the Medicare Cost Report, the Medicare Discharge File, and the MEDPAR File. The Medicare Cost Report contains the cost information that hospitals submit to fiscal intermediaries in order to be reimbursed for care provided to Medicare patients. The Medicare Discharge File indicates the number of Medicare patients admitted to a hospital in a given year. From these two sources, a national average cost per discharge is calculated.[15] The MEDPAR File is a 20 percent sample of Medicare patient bills from short-stay hospitals; this is used to create the DRG price index, which indicates the costliness of providing care for different Medicare patients in relation to the average cost per patient. Therefore, if the MEDPAR File indicates that the care of a patient in DRG 122 is 1.5 times more costly than the care of the average Medicare patient, the DRG price index is 1.5. If the national average cost per Medicare discharge is $1,000, the hospitals would be reimbursed for the care of a patient in providing service in DRG 122 at a rate of $1,000 × 1.5, or $1,500.

The DRG rate reflects the total payment for providing inpatient hospital services. In the future, the prospective payment will be updated to take into account factors such as increased costs of goods and services purchased by hospitals, improved industry productivity, and technological changes that affect specific DRGs. The rates will be considered payment in full to the hospital, except for any deductibles or co-insurance mandated by law. Hospitals are precluded from charging beneficiaries any amount that exceeds the deductible or co-insurance amounts specified by Congress.

**Phase-In Period**

Congress provided a three-year phase-in period so that hospitals have an opportunity to adjust to the prospective system (Table 2–1). In the first year of the phase-in (the fiscal year beginning October 1, 1983, and ending October 1, 1984), 75 percent of the payment rate for an individual hospital was based on the hospital's TEFRA target amount adjusted for inflation by the hospital market basket increase, plus a 1 percent technology factor. The remaining 25 percent was based on the regional DRG rate. In the second year (the fiscal year beginning October 1, 1984), 50 percent of the payment has been based on the individual hospital's TEFRA target amount adjusted for inflation by the hospital market basket increase, plus a 1 percent technology factor. The remaining 50 percent has been based on a blend of regional and national DRG rates (37.5 percent regional and 12.5 percent national).

In the third year of the phase-in (the fiscal year beginning October 1, 1985), 25 percent of the payment is to be based on the hospital's TEFRA target amount (again adjusted for inflation and technology), and the remaining 75 percent is to be based on an equal blend of regional and national DRG rates (37.5 percent each). In

**Table 2–1** Phase-In of DRG Payment Rates, 1983–1986

| Year | National Rate (%) | Regional Rate (%) | Hospital Rate (%) |
|------|------|------|------|
| 1983–1984 | | 25 | 75 |
| 1984–1985 | 12.5 | 37.5 | 50 |
| 1985–1986 | 37.5 | 37.5 | 25 |
| 1986– | 100 | | |

the fourth year (beginning October 1, 1986), 100 percent of the rate will be based on the national rate.

## Rate Calculation

The regional DRG schedules for urban and rural hospitals used during the phase-in period will be determined by the average cost per case for each of nine census divisions (Table 2–2). Furthermore, there will be an urban and a rural rate for each of the nine regions and for the nation as a whole. Thus, there will be a total of 20 DRG rates during the phase-in period.

Calculation of the reimbursable amount for a rural Alabama hospital in the third year of the DRG-based prospective payment system is shown in Table 2–3. Twenty-five percent of the DRG payment will be based on the hospital's own adjusted TEFRA target amount, 37.5 percent will be based on the rural DRG rate for the East South Central region, and 37.5 percent will be based on the rural

**Table 2–2** Adjusted Federal Standardized Payment Amounts by Census Region—Fiscal Year 1984

| | Region | Urban | Rural |
|------|--------|------|------|
| 1. | New England (CN, ME, MA, NH, RI, VT) | $2,981.03 | $2,487.26 |
| 2. | Mid-Atlantic (PA, NJ, NY) | $2,736.81 | $2,484.75 |
| 3. | South Atlantic (DE, DC, FL, GA, MD, NC, SC, VA, WV) | $2,777.47 | $2,211.96 |
| 4. | East North Central (IL, IN, MI, OH, WS) | $3,021.35 | $2,416.52 |
| 5. | East South Central (AL, KT, MS, TN) | $2,511.22 | $2,201.47 |
| 6. | West North Central (IA, KS, MN, MO, NE, ND, SD) | $2,888.76 | $2,220.88 |
| 7. | West South Central (AR, LA, OK, TX) | $2,718.88 | $2,142.45 |
| 8. | Mountain (AZ, CO, ID, MT, NV, NM, UT, WY) | $2,716.59 | $2,253.52 |
| 9. | Pacific (AK, CA, HA, OR, WA) | $2,931.40 | $2,406.80 |
| 10. | National | $2,837.91 | $2,264.00 |

*Source: Federal Register*, Vol. 48, September 1, 1983, pp. 39,763 and 39,844.

**Table 2–3** Computation of Payment for a Rural Alabama Hospital in the Third Year

*Payment* = 0.25 (Hospital-Specific Rate) + 0.375 (Regional Rate, Rural) + 0.375 (National Rate, Rural)

| P = 0.25 [(Cost per Case) | (DRG Index)] | + 0.375 [(Cost per Case) | (DRG Index)] | + 0.375 [(Cost per Case) | (DRG Index)] |
|---|---|---|---|---|---|
| Base year adjusted by hospital market basket factor and medical technology factor | From MEDPAR File | Base year adjusted by change in actual costs from prior year, hospital market basket factor, medical technology factor, and area wages | From MEDPAR File | Base year adjusted by change in actual costs from prior year, hospital market basket factor, medical technology factor, and national rural wages | From MEDPAR File |

*Note:*  Cost per case amounts do not include capital costs and medical education costs.

national DRG rate. In the fourth year, the payment rate for this hospital will be based entirely on the rural national rate adjusted for area wages.

The hospital-specific cost per case used during the phase-in period will reflect the hospital's own cost per case in the base year (October 1, 1981 to September 30, 1982). The base year cost per case will be computed from Medicare allowable costs, excluding capital costs and medical education costs. These costs will be considered "pass throughs," and hospitals will be reimbursed for them separately. After the first year, the hospital-specific cost-per-case amount is computed by adjusting the base year cost per case to take into account the rate of increase in the hospital market basket between the base year and the prospective year, plus an allowance for technology.

The regional cost per case is projected from the base year of 1981 adjusted for the increase in actual costs between 1981 and 1982, the rate of increase in the hospital market basket between 1983 and 1984, and an allowance for medical technology. The national rates will be based on the national average cost per case from the base year, with adjustments for the same rate factors used to project regional prices.

Table 2–4 shows in general how to calculate the payment rate for DRG 125 for an urban hospital in the West South Central Region for the first three years of the plan. The target percent is assumed to be 6 percent in the last two years, and the same wage index is used each year. Adjustments for budget neutrality and outlier payments after 1984 are ignored. The data show this hospital's payment for DRG 125 will rise from $4,787 to $5,530, a gain of 15.5 percent over the two-year period from fiscal year 1984 to fiscal year 1986. Thus, the payment rate will rise at a much faster rate than the compounded target percentage increase (12.4 percent). The difference stems from the changing weights (hospital-specific, regional, and national) and the fact that the hospital's DRG-specific cost base is below the standardized DRG payment amount. If the opposite were true, the payment rates could decrease over time, even with a positive inflation adjustment.

## Adjustments

Hospitals will be reimbursed for direct medical costs on a reasonable cost basis during the phase-in period (until October 1, 1986). Recognizing that hospitals with medical education programs have higher costs, Congress provided for retrospective reimbursement of direct expenses, such as salaries of interns and residents.[16] Hospitals may receive additional payments for their indirect education costs, such as extra tests ordered by residents and research costs.[17] Hospitals will not be reimbursed for indirect costs as they are reimbursed for direct medical education costs, however. Instead, for every 0.1 increase in the hospital's ratio of interns and residents to hospital beds, there will be a 12.12 percent increase in the

**Table 2–4** Calculation of Payment Rate for DRG 125, Urban Hospital X, West South Central Region: Fiscal Years (FYs) 1984–1986 (Rounded in Dollars)

| Component | FY 1984 | FY 1985 | FY 1986 |
|---|---|---|---|
| Hospital portion: | | | |
| Adjusted base year cost | $3,096 | $3,096 | $3,096 |
| Case mix index | ÷1.07 | ÷1.07 | ÷1.07 |
| | $2,893 | $2,893 | $2,893 |
| Target percent | * | ×1.06 | ×1.124 |
| | $2,893 | $3,067 | $3,252 |
| DRG weight | ×1.6455 | ×1.6455 | ×1.6455 |
| | $4,760 | $5,047 | $5,351 |
| Hospital percent | ×.75 | ×.50 | ×.25 |
| Hospital amount | $3,570 | $2,524 | $1,338 |
| Regional portion: | | | |
| Standard amount for labor-related items | $2,146 | $2,146 | $2,146 |
| Wage index | ×1.1119 | ×1.1119 | ×1.1119 |
| | $2,386 | $2,386 | $2,386 |
| Standard amount for non-labor-related items | +$573 | +$573 | +$573 |
| | $2,959 | $2,959 | $2,959 |
| Target percent | * | ×1.06 | ×1.124 |
| | $2,959 | $3,137 | $3,326 |
| DRG weight | ×1.6455 | ×1.6455 | ×1.6455 |
| | $4,869 | $5,162 | $5,473 |
| Regional percent | ×.25 | ×.375 | ×.375 |
| Regional amount | $1,217 | $1,936 | $2,052 |
| National portion: | | | |
| Standard amount for labor-related items | $2,206 | $2,206 | $2,206 |
| Wage index | ×1.1119 | ×1.1119 | ×1.1119 |
| | $2,453 | $2,453 | $2,453 |
| Standard amount for non-labor-related items | +$632 | +$632 | +$632 |
| | $3,085 | $3,085 | $3,085 |
| Target percent | * | ×1.06 | ×1.124 |
| | $3,085 | $3,270 | $3,468 |
| DRG weight | ×1.6455 | ×1.6455 | ×1.6455 |
| | $5,076 | $5,381 | $5,707 |
| National percent | ×.00 | ×.125 | ×.375 |
| National amount | $ 0 | $ 673 | $2,140 |
| Total payment rate | $4,787 | $5,133 | $5,530 |

Note: *Base year costs are updated through FY 1984. Target percent equals inflation plus one percentage point per year.

Source: Reprinted with permission from *Hospital Progress*, October 1983. Copyright 1983 by the Catholic Health Association.

DRG rate. Congress raised the adjustment to this level after hearing testimony that the percentage adjustment under TEFRA was inadequate.

Although capital costs will be passed through retrospectively during the phase-in period, the secretary of HHS submitted a report to Congress in October 1984 on the ways in which capital costs can be included in the prospective payment system. If no legislation concerning capital costs has been enacted by October 1, 1986, Medicare may refuse to pay for capital expenditures after that date unless they have been approved by a state review program.

Hospitals also have a safety mechanism available for patients who require excessively expensive care or excessively long lengths of stay. These patients are referred to as "outliers." The legislation directs the secretary to develop payment rates for the marginal cost of care beyond certain "cut-off points." These payment rates are applicable only when a patient's length of stay exceeds the mean length of stay for the DRG by a fixed number of days or by a fixed number of standard deviations. A hospital may also request additional payments for patients whose costs are a "fixed multiple" of the average cost of providing care to patients in the DRG to which the patient is assigned. Payments for outlier care will equal the DRG payment plus payments to cover the "marginal costs" of the days beyond the cut-off point. Marginal payment rates for outliers will be paid only if the Health Care Financing Administration (HCFA) grants a special request from a hospital for additional payment. Only 5 to 6 percent of DRG-related Medicare expenditures may be used to make supplemental payments for "outlier" cases, however, and these payments can be adjusted from year to year to ensure that the total amount of outlier payments remains within the mandated limit.

Congress also authorized adjustments for regional and national referral centers and hospitals that serve a disproportionate number of low-income or Medicare patients. The way in which these adjustments will be made and the requirements a hospital must meet to qualify for them are not specified in the legislation, but will probably be spelled out in the regulations.[18]

These adjustments for medical education costs, capital costs, outliers, and costs associated with serving disproportionate numbers of low-income patients appear to provide hospitals with ample opportunity to increase their revenues. The "budget neutrality" clause mandates, however, that total Medicare expenditures under the prospective system for fiscal years 1984 and 1985 cannot exceed those that would have been made on the basis of the target amounts under TEFRA. Thus, the secretary can adjust the standardized DRG rates and outlier payments downward as needed to meet this requirement.[19]

The legislation provides hospitals with a right to administrative or judicial review of computational errors, exceptions, and adjustments. Congress has prohibited any such review of adjustments to maintain budget neutrality, of the use of DRGs, of the way patients are classified into DRGs, or of the use of DRG cost weights, however.

States that have a prospective payment system applicable to all payers may be exempted from the federal payment system, provided that certain conditions are met. Alternate prospective payment systems may also be substituted for Medicare prospective payment if the program has state approval, applies to at least 75 percent of all revenue, does not increase Medicare expenditures, and does not impede access to care.[20]

## MANAGEMENT CONCERNS AND POTENTIAL PROBLEMS

The Medicare prospective payment system has been designed to evolve over time in response to provider and congressional concerns. The secretary of HHS has been directed to provide certain reports, experiments, and demonstration projects in order to refine the present system. These requirements are indications of possible congressional actions in the future (Table 2–5).

Other issues have not yet been formally considered by Congress. For example, since DRGs do not reflect the severity of illness within a given DRG, researchers at Johns Hopkins University are advocating the use of a severity index to take into account disease stages, recovery rates, remission of acute symptoms, complications, preexisting conditions, and the effect of non–operating room procedures on the utilization of hospital resources.[21] Others have proposed that each physician be required to reimburse hospitals for the services rendered to his or her patients and, in turn, be allowed to realize financial dividends for cost-effective care.[22] The same concept could be applied in a system that provided for hospital payments to physicians for inpatient services. In addition, care provided in an outpatient setting may eventually be included in a prospective payment system;[23] the result may be prospective reimbursement for a specific service *regardless* of the health care setting.

Predictions about the ultimate action (if any) on these reports and proposals are speculative. Consequently, hospital administrators must live with a great deal of uncertainty and an unstable environment in the foreseeable future.

### Cost Shifting

Since prospective reimbursement presently applies only to Medicare patients and selected private plans in selected areas, some hospitals may attempt to compensate for the losses from restrictive Medicare payments by increasing charges in departments that have a low rate of utilization by Medicare patients and a high rate of utilization by privately insured patients. Because of this enormous potential for cost shifting, most observers expect all payment systems to become prospective in the future.

**Table 2–5** Partial Listing of Required HHS Reports to Congress

| Subject | Date Due | Requirements |
|---|---|---|
| Impact of prospective payment system | Annual reports from fiscal year 1984 to fiscal year 1987 | Impact of prospective payment system on hospitals, beneficiaries, and other payers; evaluation of regional vs. national payment rates |
| Capital prospective payment system | October 20, 1984 | Provisions for including capital-related costs, such as return on net equity, interests, and depreciation in the prospective payment system |
| Uncompensated care costs | April 1, 1985 | Provisions for including uncompensated care allowances |
| Cost information | April 1, 1985 | Feasibility of requiring hospitals to provide cost of care information to both public and private payers |
| Physician inclusion | Data collection to begin in fiscal year 1984; report due in fiscal year 1985 | Feasibility of setting prospective DRG rates on inpatient physician services |
| Refinements to prospective payment system | 1985 annual report | Impact of eliminating urban vs. rural differential, development of prospective payment for exempt hospitals and units, modifications to address outliers and severity of illness issues, impact on cost shifting, and the advisability of extending system to all payers |
| Recalibration of DRGs | 1986 | Recalibration of relative weights of DRGs |

In the meantime, it is extremely difficult for an individual hospital to develop an integrated cost control strategy. There are incentives for cost control only for the care of Medicare patients; Blue Cross and other commercial payers continue to reward hospitals financially for using more bed days and ancillary services. With such diverse payment practices among payers, some hospitals may respond to the payment environment by turning to accountants and lawyers, rather than by improving management systems and physician utilization practices. Thus, success of the prospective reimbursement could be jeopardized, not because it is an ineffective payment system, but because the confused incentives in the system do not provide clear goals for the hospital and medical communities.

To avoid cost shifting, commercial insurers will begin to implement prospective payment mechanisms that are identical or similar to those found in the Medicare program. This will make it necessary for hospitals to improve their management efficiency, since they will be unable to recover losses through cost shifting.[24]

The Health Insurance Association of America has lobbied strongly for the prospective payment system to cover all payers. Without a prospective payment system, this group estimates that cost shifting to the private sector could reach $12 billion by 1985.[25] Senator Edward M. Kennedy has proposed legislation to encourage states to develop their own prospective payment plans for all third party payers.

## Validity of the Payment Schedule

Several studies in recent years have questioned the validity of the data on which the DRG prospective payment system is based. One study noted that "there is as yet no taxonomy based on clinical data that can demonstrably classify cases in terms of their severity and clinical case management into a set of exhaustive and mutually exclusive homogeneous cells."[26] Furthermore, there is as yet neither a theoretical base nor empirical evidence to indicate that DRGs contain only cases whose clinically optimal management requires highly similar resource costs.[27]

Because the DRG categories have not been developed within a conceptual framework that incorporates quality of care, the empirically derived categories result from averaging well-treated with ill-treated cases. Moreover, the classification systems have been developed from multi-institutional data bases that vary in terms of quality, clinical appropriateness, and resource availability.[28]

Since little is known about the relationship between cost and quality, their simultaneous control by a single mechanism, such as prospective reimbursement, may not be a realistic goal. The choice appears to be between a system that imposes constraints, probably without quality-enhancing incentives, and one that does not. As Berki pointed out,

> The fundamental problem here is that we do not know whether the "recipes" are correct or not; they have not been pretested. Measures of service bundles have been derived from observing limited sets of hospitals without any explicit clinical quality standards. The recipes, the measures of mean services per case, and hence their associated charges, repeat what the average cook does, the average of the excellent and the poor, the efficient and the wasteful. Payment schemes which have desirable incentive characteristics, should not be based on the average of the system as a whole but on the performance of institutions whose clinical and economic performance meets appropriate quality of care and efficiency levels.[29]

Other authors have also concluded that the DRG categories are based on inadequate and invalid data. Some of the data were concurrent, while other data were retrospective; yet, there seems to be a wide discrepancy in how patients are classified initially (concurrent) and at discharge (retrospective).[30] Moreover, the data being used by the HCFA probably do not fully reflect the level of care complexity. This lack of homogeneity within DRG categories has also been noted in the New Jersey experiment with prospective reimbursement based on DRGs.[31] Consequently, reimbursement based on that data may be incorrect.[32]

An individual hospital's DRG-specific adjusted actual costs per case will almost certainly differ from the national average costs for that DRG. Cost inefficiency is one possible explanation, but the wide disparity in the medical problems besetting patients in most DRGs may be a contributing factor.[33]

This disparity occurs because the DRGs do not take into account the severity of the medical problem, do not recognize more than one complication, and provide inadequate adjustments for a patient's age. Diggs felt that DRGs are not predictive of actual hospital costs because of their failure to account for the patient's intensity of illness.[34] As a result, hospitals will be inadequately reimbursed. For example, some urban public general hospitals admit mostly high-risk obstetrical patients who require intensive services. In Diggs' view, nonweighted classification systems do not fit hospitals in which each patient is given a customized diagnosis and treatment.

The data on which the DRG payments are based have also been called into question. When Doremus and Michenzi compared data from the MEDPAR file, the original medical record discharge orders, and reabstracted records for University Hospital in Cleveland, they found widely divergent diagnostic and surgical data that resulted in significant variations in DRG classification and reimbursement.[35] Specifically, the use of data from the MEDPAR file led to a considerably lower level of Medicare reimbursement. Moreover, the diagnostic and surgical information in the medical record was inaccurate and incomplete because of human error and basic differences in opinion among those processing the data. Only the case mix index calculated from reabstracted record information was considered reliable, because greater care was taken during the reabstracting coding process.

One recent study showed that the claims data (MEDPAR file) used by the HCFA to assess hospital case mix were inaccurate (or inadequate) an average of 50 percent of the time.[36] This error resulted in an average understatement in hospital case mix and reimbursement of about 4 percent of the figures calculated from more accurate and complete medical record data. Thus, the HCFA's use of this inadequate data base alone may cost the average hospital about $300,000 per year and will cost the larger tertiary care hospitals with more complex cases substantially more.

There has also been some criticism of the data used to adjust DRG rates. For example, hospitals say that the regional wage index is riddled with inaccuracies. The index was calculated by dividing hospitals' total salary expenditures by their number of employees. No distinction was made, however, between full-time employees earning a full salary and part-time employees earning much less.[37] Therefore, the index for rural hospitals, which use many part-time employees, may be artificially low.

Many hospital administrators believe that arbitrary distinctions, such as geographical boundaries, may have a greater effect on reimbursement levels under the new payment system than does good management.[38] Hospitals that are just inside or just outside a geographical boundary may suffer as a result of the regional wage index adjustment. All hospitals in a state that fall outside a designated urban area are considered nonurban and assigned a rural wage index. This could be a problem for a "rural" hospital that borders an urban area and competes in the same labor market, since its reimbursement would not reflect this fact.

As a result of these data problems, the typical hospital will probably be overpaid or underpaid under DRG-based reimbursement. Nevertheless, the critical issue is whether overages and underages cancel each other. While a balance of overages and underages is unlikely in a given year, the differences may not be statistically significant. Whether there will be significant differences over time for a given hospital is unknown, however.

## DRG Creep

The deliberate and systematic shift in a hospital's reported case mix in order to improve reimbursement is referred to as DRG creep.[39] Since category assignment is partially dependent on the nature of the secondary and tertiary diagnoses recorded, a simple change in the order of their coding not only may upgrade a case into a higher cost category, but also may increase the numerical value of the case mix. Simborg concluded that, by switching the first and second diagnoses, and by selecting the costlier of two possible DRGs for each discharge, the University of California at San Francisco Hospital could have increased the cost of its case mix index by 14 percent.[40] Such "editing" of discharge abstracts would have resulted in an unprecedented windfall profit for the hospital. Although the number of incorrectly reported principal diagnoses would be increased, the increase might not be noted since the base line error rate is normally so high.

The informal process by which physicians learn from experience and adjust their practice accordingly could also contribute to DRG creep. There are legitimate medical vagaries and uncertainties in many diagnostic situations, and it is not always easy to determine when a less costly DRG becomes a more costly DRG. Minor diagnostic nuances and slight imprecisions of wording have little clinical importance, yet they have major financial consequences under DRG-based reimbursement. Because reimbursement for various services is tied to the vagaries, uncertainties, subtleties, and errors of discharge, the potential for DRG creep is high and may have serious adverse effects on the entire cost containment effort. There will be strong incentives to look a little harder and to perform that extra test or procedure to make a diagnosis.

In order to forestall DRG creep, the HCFA expects to audit approximately 20 to 25 percent of the bills submitted by hospitals under the prospective payment system.[41] Grimaldi noted that this type of scrutiny is likely to identify and deter incorrect sequencing. Moreover, the ethical implications will dissuade medical records personnel from dishonest sequencing.[42] Finally, long-term financial consequences of improper coding may overpower short-term gains if upcoding today produces inadequate reimbursement tomorrow; cases reported as more complex will appear less costly to the hospital than those that are truly more complex as HCFA adjusts its DRG prices to reflect new information. The result may be inadequate reimbursement in the long run.

### Physician-Administrator Relations

The prospective payment system includes no direct incentives to control physicians' practice patterns. Hospitals do not necessarily control the physicians on their staffs; yet physician involvement in the management of patient services is essential because hospitals are at risk for factors such as length of stay, use and volume of ancillary services, and patient mix.

Before the implementation of DRG-based reimbursement, the work of physicians increased gross revenues and total reimbursement to the hospital. Under the new system, however, physicians' activities will "consume money."[43] This change in the reimbursement system is directed toward containing hospital costs, but not physician charges. The current structure of the DRG payment system does not contain incentives for physicians to be cost-efficient.[44] To the contrary, physicians' income will increase with additional ancillary services, tests, and treatments, as well as longer lengths of stay.[45] Physicians will therefore derive short-term benefits by maintaining the traditional treatment patterns, but these inefficient treatment patterns will cause financial solvency problems for the hospital. Since Congress has implemented a plan that places physicians and hospitals in an adversarial relationship, good communications and cooperation between hospital management and physicians are imperative. Otherwise, the survival of the hospital could be threatened.

### Impact on Quality of Care

As Studnicki has pointed out, any new government- or industry-sponsored policy initiatives in the health care arena will have unanticipated consequences.[46]

On one hand, the hospital must serve the needs of its various constituencies (e.g., physicians, patients, researchers, and students) who are all concerned with the "quality" of care, but who define it in somewhat different ways. On the other hand, the hospital is an economic entity seeking to increase its financial stability and improve its ability to survive. The new legislation fosters the assumption that efforts to control costs through prospective payment will have little or no effect on the achievement of other objectives, such as quality.[47] In reality, there is a strong possibility that DRG payments will provide financial incentives to distort the legitimate practice of medical art and science.

### Communication with Staff and the General Public

In addition to educating physicians in the realities of the new payment system, hospital administrators must help other staff members and the general public to understand the system. Many hospitals have prepared video presentations on prospective payment to be shown to all employees.[48] Attendance at workshops and staff retreats are other methods used to communicate the intricacies of the new system to staff. The public is concerned about the impact of DRGs on access to high-quality care. Medicare beneficiaries may fear that physicians will refuse to treat them, and private paying patients may fear that hospitals will shift more cost to them. In order to solve these potential problems, hospitals must have an active program of communication with the staff and with the general public.

### Hospital Survival

Some rural hospital administrators fear that their institutions, which perform less complicated and less costly procedures than do larger urban hospitals, could collapse under the new payment system.[49] As they see it, the present urban-rural differentials overcompensate for the true cost differentials; they favor a national average payment scheme.

Ultimately, the prospective payment system could drive up hospital costs in rural areas.[50] If rural hospitals cannot afford to modernize, many specialists will return to urban medical centers. Rural patients will then have to seek care at more expensive and harder to reach metropolitan hospitals. As small, rural hospitals lose these patients, they may have to increase the rates for remaining patients in order to cover their fixed costs.

On the other hand, some administrators of urban hospitals claim that their hospitals are being shortchanged under the new system.[51] In particular, they are concerned that the DRG payment rates fail to take into account the urban hospital's provision of services to the indigent. While the New Jersey prospective payment system did include an adjustment for the care of low-income patients, Congress did not include such an adjustment in the 1983 federal legislation. Urban hospitals also claim that they have almost twice as many outliers as do hospitals nationwide.

Aside from which types of hospitals will benefit or suffer under the new payment schedule, the present and future adequacy of Medicare payments to hospitals has caused some concern. The payment rates are much lower than many administrators had anticipated, thus resulting in revenue shortfalls.[52] On June 18, 1984, HHS announced that 1985 Medicare prospective payment rate increases would be only 5.6 percent over 1984 levels, adding that average per case payments would actually be 6 percent over 1984 projections because of other changes. This is the lowest rate of increase since Medicare began in 1965.

Empirical evidence suggests that the New Jersey prospective payment program reduced the rate of increase in hospital expenditures per day and per admission.[53,54] It may have succeeded in containing costs at the expense of the financial viability of regulated hospitals, however.[55] The financial position of the average New Jersey hospital has deteriorated more than the national average since the enactment of that state's program. Moreover, inner city, urban, and teaching hospitals were affected more than suburban hospitals were affected, probably because suburban hospitals were able to transfer more costs to patients with private insurance, since such patients are more prevalent in suburban hospitals.[56] Such a deterioration in their financial position may force institutions to defer the maintenance of existing plant assets and to use capital reserves to finance operations.[57] Thus, the service life of existing plant assets would be shortened and the institution's ability to replace capital equipment eroded.

## POTENTIAL BENEFITS

Despite the problems and potential problems, the advantages of the new prospective payment system should outweigh the disadvantages in the long run. Adjustments will be made if and when major problems with the original legislation and regulatory guidelines become apparent. This does not mean, however, that benefits will exceed costs for any individual hospital—there will be winners and losers.

The prospective payment system will promote efficiency and cost containment by allowing hospitals to retain any surplus that they can earn by operating efficiently (or by other methods). The prospective payment system should also improve the quality of inpatient care by encouraging hospitals to specialize in the services that they perform best. In general, infrequently performed services are associated with a lower quality of care. Finally, a national evaluation of state rate-setting programs has shown that prospective payment has no adverse effect on hospital accreditation status, mortality rates, readmission rates, or other quality indexes.[58]

According to former secretary of HHS Schweiker, the new system has several other advantages:[59]

1. It has been implemented quickly.
2. It ensures both hospitals and the federal government of a predictable payment for services.
3. It reduces the administrative burden on hospitals and provides rewards for hospital administrators to operate efficiently. The President's Private Sector Survey on Cost Control projected that these rewards for efficiency would save the government more than $13 billion from 1984 through 1986.[60]
4. It can result in improved quality of care as hospitals begin to specialize in what they do best.
5. Medicare patient liability will be limited to the co-insurance and deductible payments mandated by Congress.

Whether all these alleged advantages and benefits are achieved remains to be seen. Given the deficiencies of the old retrospective system, however, evolution of a prospective payment system seems inevitable.

---

**NOTES**

1. Richard S. Schweiker, *Report to Congress: Hospital Prospective Payment for Medicare* (Washington, D.C.: U.S. Department of Health and Human Services, 1982), 3.

2. John K. Inglehart, "The New Era of Prospective Payment for Hospitals," *New England Journal of Medicine* 307 (November 11, 1982): 1288.

3. James D. Bentley and Peter W. Butler, "Measurement of Case Mix," *Topics in Health Care Financing* 8 (Summer 1982): 1–11.

4. Paul L. Grimaldi and Julie A. Micheletti, *Diagnosis Related Groups: A Practitioner's Guide* (Chicago: Pluribus Press, 1982), 18.

5. Martin Feldstein, *Economic Analysis for Health Service Efficiency* (Chicago: Markham, 1968).

6. Leonard Goodisman and Tom Trompeter, "Hospital Case Mix and Average Charge per Case: An Initial Study," *Health Services Research* 14 (Spring 1979): 44–55.

7. Grimaldi and Micheletti, *A Practitioner's Guide.*

8. Paul L. Grimaldi and Julie A. Micheletti, "Homogeneity Revisited: The New DRG's," *Journal of the American Medical Records Association* 53 (April 1982): 56.

9. Walter P. Wood, Richard P. Ament, and Edward J. Kobinoki, "A Foundation for Hospital Case Mix Management," *Inquiry* 18 (Fall 1981): 247–254.

10. Grimaldi and Micheletti, "Homogeneity Revisited."

11. Leo K. Lichtig, "Data Systems for Case Mix," *Topics in Health Care Financing* 8 (Summer 1982): 13–19.

12. Paul L. Grimaldi, "The Physician and the DRG Model," *Journal of the Medical Society of New Jersey* 77 (April 1980): 279–281.

13. Grimaldi and Micheletti, "Homogeneity Revisited."

14. Ernst and Whinney, *The Social Security Amendments of 1983, Title 6* (Chicago: Ernst and Whinney, 1983).

15. Schweiker, *Hospital Prospective Payment for Medicare.*

16. Ernst and Whinney, *The Revised DRGs: Their Importance in Medicare Payments to Hospitals* (Chicago: Ernst and Whinney, 1983).

17. Ibid.

18. Ibid.

19. Ibid.

20. American Hospital Association, *Medicare Prospective Pricing: Legislative Summary and Management Implications* (Washington, D.C.: American Hospital Association, 1983).

21. "Severity Index Applied to DRGs Accounts for Sicker Patients," *Hospitals* 56 (December 16, 1982): 37.

22. Thomas E. McKeown, "Better Yet, Have Them Pay the Bills," *Healthcare Financial Management* 3 (January 1983): 37.

23. Schweiker, *Hospital Prospective Payment for Medicare.*

24. David Lefton, "Caution, Support in Testimony on DRG Prospective Pay Plan," *American Medical News* 26 (March 4, 1983): 2–8.

25. "HIAA Ad Pushes All-Payer Prospective Pay Alternatives," *Modern Healthcare* 13 (April 1983): 29.

26. Wanda W. Young, Robert B. Swinkola, and Dorothy M. Zorn, "The Measurement of Hospital Case Mix," *Medical Care* 20 (April 1982): 501.

27. Richard P. Ament, James L. Dreachslin, Edward J. Kobrinski, and Walter R. Wood, "Three Case-Type Classifications: Suitability for Use in Reimbursing Hospitals," *Medical Care* 20 (April 1982): 460.

28. S.E. Berki, "The Design of Case-Based Hospital Payment Systems," *Medical Care* 21 (January 1983): 1–13.

29. Ibid., 7–8.

30. Cynthia Barnard and Truman Esmond, "DRG-Based Reimbursement: The Use of Concurrent and Retrospective Clinical Data," *Medical Care* 19 (November 1981): 1071–1082.

31. Robert H. Davies and George Westfall, "Reimbursement under DRG's: Implementation in New Jersey," *Health Services Research* 18 (Summer 1983): 233–244.

32. Barnard and Esmond, "DRG-Based Reimbursement."

33. Grimaldi and Micheletti, "Homogeneity Revisited."

34. "Lack of Intensity of Illness Factor Causes DRG's To Predict Inaccurate Hospital Costs," *Hospitals* 56 (May 16, 1982): 54.

35. Harvey D. Doremus and Elana M. Michenzi, "Data Quality: An Illustration of Its Potential Impact upon Diagnosis-Related Group's Case Mix Index and Reimbursement," *Medical Care* 21 (October 1983): 1001–1011.

36. Ibid.

37. "No Major Changes Seen in Final Regs," *Modern Healthcare* 13 (December 1983): 23–28.

38. Michele L. Robinson and Cynthia Wallace, "Who Wins or Loses under Prospective Pay? The Decision Could Be Arbitrary," *Modern Healthcare* 13 (October 1983): 46–54.

39. Donald W. Simborg, "DRG Creep: A New Hospital-Acquired Disease," *New England Journal of Medicine* 304 (June 25, 1981): 1602–1604.

40. Ibid.

41. "HCFA To Audit Up to 25 Percent of Hospital PRS Bills," *Hospitals* 57 (November 16, 1983): 24.

42. Paul L. Grimaldi, "DRG Reimbursement in New Jersey: Some Initial Results," *Hospital Progress* 62 (January 1981): 41–46.

43. Emily Friedman, "Getting to Know Us: Hospitals May Finally Learn about True Cost and Pricing," *Hospitals* 57 (March 16, 1983): 74–82.

44. Thomas G. Dehn and Karen M. Sandrich, *What Doctors Should Know about DRGs* (Chicago: Care Communications, 1983).

45. Lynn Kahn, "Meeting of the Minds: Hospital-Physician Diplomacy Crucial under Prospective Reimbursement," *Hospitals* 57 (April 1983): 84–86.

46. James Studnicki, "Regulation by DRG: Policy or Perversion?" *Hospital and Health Services Administration* 28 (January-February 1983): 96–110.

47. Ibid.

48. Cynthia Wallace, "Hospitals Will Be Shooting in the Dark after Prospective Pay Bill Okd," *Modern Healthcare* 13 (May 1983): 18.

49. Linda Punch, "Rural Units May Topple under New Payment Plan," *Modern Healthcare* 13 (April 1983): 20.

50. Ibid.

51. "Urban Hospitals Cite PPS Drawbacks," *Hospitals* 57 (November 1, 1983): 24.

52. Michele L. Robinson, "Low Prospective Payment Rates May Surprise Some Administrators," *Modern Healthcare* 13 (September 1983): 24–26.

53. Craig Coelen and Daniel Sullivan, "An Analysis of the Effects of Prospective Reimbursement Programs on Hospital Expenditures," *Health Care Financing Review* 2 (Winter 1981): 1–40.

54. Michael D. Rosco, "Impact of Prospective Rate Setting on Hospital Expenditures and Financial Position," Paper Presented at the American Public Health Association Annual Meeting, November 6, 1982.

55. Michael D. Rosco and Robert W. Broyles, "Unintended Consequences of Prospective Payment: Erosion of Hospital Financial Position and Cost Shifting," *Health Care Management Review* 9 (Summer 1984): 35–43.

56. Nancy Worthington, Jerry Cromwell, Gilbey Kamens, and James Kanak, "Case Study of Prospective Reimbursement in New Jersey," in *Health Care Financing Contracts and Grants Report: National Hospital Rate Setting Study*, vol. 6 (Baltimore: U.S. Department of Health, Education, and Welfare, Health Care Financing Administration, April 1980).

57. Rosco and Broyles, "Unintended Consequences."

58. Richard S. Schweiker, "Executive Summary of Report to Congress on Hospital Prospective Payment for Medicare," *Healthcare Financial Management* 3 (March 1983): 67–69.

59. Ibid.

60. "Prospective Pricing Will Bring Savings," *Hospitals* 57 (June 1, 1983): 23.

# Chapter 3

# Strategic Factors: Planning

Amid the turmoil generated by Medicare's shift to a reimbursement plan based on diagnosis-related groups (DRGs) and emulations by other third party payers, hospital executives have become aware that their environment has changed dramatically. Despite the confusion surrounding these changes, specific management plans must be articulated. Thus, although DRG-based reimbursement will have a profound influence on third party payers, physicians, ancillary staff, and patients, the greatest effect will be felt by hospital executives.

Because they are ultimately responsible to the governing board for fiscal performance, hospital executives must translate prospective payments into effective strategic plans, operating policies, and standardized procedures. It is a question of modifying the strategic plans and internal operations of hospitals to manage the ensuing change most effectively. The sooner hospital executives begin to create the necessary management strategies, the sooner they will be able to guide medical and ancillary staff members toward a position that is mutually beneficial to them and to the hospital.

## HOSPITAL PLANNING PROBLEMS

In the past, hospitals have often been reluctant to make a sincere commitment to planning. Failure to plan, however, results in few definitive actions for the short run and little practical guidance for the long run.

There are many reasons and excuses given for overlooking planning activities as a daily management response. For example, the daily press of decisions, meetings, communications, and unexpected events that seem to demand immediate attention consumes the present. This makes it difficult to allocate sufficient time to the planning function. The forces of distraction are strong, because it is more glamorous and exciting to manage current issues than to plan for the future. There is an urgency associated with current decisions that reinforces the behavior of executives who are always fighting fires.

The lack of foresight—analysis and forecasting—in hospital executives also inhibits planning. Executives seldom devote sufficient time to identifying the information that they will need to make better decisions and plan. Thus, they may reach a critical decision point only to discover that they do not have precise and accurate information. Planning for the future requires executives to consider the types of decisions that must be made over the long run.

The rapid advancement and the proliferation of medical technology present serious challenges to hospitals and further complicate the planning task. On one hand, hospitals want to have only the finest equipment with the greatest productivity in order to provide high-quality care while meeting economic goals. On the other hand, it is very expensive to change equipment continually, especially when the economic life of a product has not been fully exhausted. With the high capital investment required for some radiological equipment, for example, it may be best to forego equipment replacement until there has been a return on the initial investment. Clearly, given the magnitude of capital involved in these decisions, hospital executives can seldom justify a failure to plan for them.

Finally, hospital executives simply may not know how to plan. They may not have sufficient knowledge or experience to

- establish a hierarchy of meaningful missions, aims, goals, and objectives
- formulate operational strategies and tactics
- integrate planning and control in order to ensure that objectives are accomplished
- instill commitment to the planning function in medical and nonmedical staff members
- structure the planning process to ensure that all operating levels in the hospital have input into the formation of goals and objectives
- reinforce individuals and departments for accomplishing their goals and objectives
- penalize individuals and departments for failing to accomplish their intended results
- develop a vision of the hospital's potential progress, given the resources at its disposal and the context in which it exists

## PLANNING FOR PROSPECTIVE REIMBURSEMENT

The implementation of prospective reimbursement will require hospital executives to analyze very carefully the mission of hospitals and the strategies that can be used to guide them toward formally defined ends. It will also necessitate consideration of the best way to implement plans with the medical and support departments of the hospital. Prospective payment, therefore, is a challenge that will test the very best hospital executive. Effective management of prospective payment systems requires a sophisticated, timely, and operationally viable planning system.

In this sense, prospective payment may help to accomplish more than just cost containment in hospitals. It may also stimulate improved planning within hospitals. Hospitals in which the planning function is already established and operationally refined may find it easier to begin planning for prospective payment, but the gradual introduction of DRGs by Medicare provides at least some lead time for hospitals that have seriously neglected planning in the past to begin planning for the new system.

## Use of Consultants

Many hospitals will avail themselves of consultants to undertake this sort of planning for them. The use of consultants in forming plans for prospective payment, however, suggests that the hospital has little confidence in its ability to come to grips with a major environmental change. It also suggests that the planning process has been neglected in the past.

Hospital executives should develop confidence in their own ability to plan and to ascertain the appropriate direction to pursue in light of major environmental changes, such as prospective reimbursement. They should be philosophically prepared to meet whatever challenge the future brings. It is precisely this mind set that differentiates effective managers from ineffective managers. Effective managers are conceptually committed to planning and are therefore prepared to institute new planning that may increase their hospital's benefits from prospective payment.

Although consultants should not be used as a substitute for rigorous thinking and effective action on the part of hospital executives, they can and possibly should be used to verify the strategies and tactics that hospital executives have already formulated in response to DRGs or prospective payment. Consultants can validate the efficacy of planning decisions, the choice of one action over another, the tactics used to achieve objectives, or even the overall direction of a hospital if certain milestones are reached. Consultants can also be used to inject fresh, innovative alternatives into the planning process.

In regard to planning for DRG-based reimbursement, the emphasis should be on obtaining advice from consultants rather than relying on them to manage every aspect of the new system. If a hospital discovers that it must rely excessively on external consultants, it may need a wholesale change in the management team.

Consultants can offer good advice, but they cannot replace the management expertise of the full-time staff.

## Importance of Environmental Monitoring

The decision to plan, or to modify existing plans, in response to the implementation of prospective payment is consistent with the well-established management principle that there is a direct association between a hospital and its environment. With the growth of systems analysis in the 1950s and 1960s, it was recognized that hospitals, like other organizations, must deliberately modify their internal processes if they expect to attain the highest levels of performance. Hospital executives can no longer view their organizations as relatively immune to the forces that surround them.

The idea that hospital executives should better monitor their environment may be more complex than it first appears. Hospital executives must consider, for example, the magnitude of current environmental changes and the direction that hospitals will take over the next ten years in view of those changes. Any changes in Medicaid or private insurer coverage must be carefully monitored by hospitals and integrated with parallel changes in Medicare. The specifics of these changes are always important in hospital functioning, but the changes may have even greater importance for strategic planning.

Clearly, the content and the intended results of plans must capture the very essence of the existing *and* the future environment. In operational terms, this means that hospitals should incorporate the developments in prospective payment by third party payers into their goals and objectives, as well as into their strategies and tactics to achieve these goals and objectives. For example, if the prospective payment system under Medicare indicates that a hospital's average length of stay will decrease and its outpatient services will increase, it would accomplish little for that hospital to continue pre-DRG planning for bed expansion; the facilities that may be needed most in the immediate future (i.e., the next three to five years) are outpatient facilities.

Particularly germane is the extent to which prospective payment systems will affect a hospital's capital expenditures. Facilities and the services provided in these facilities must be carefully planned well in advance to arrange the necessary financing and to procure the quality in design and construction that make the project worthwhile. Hospitals are in a predicament in this regard, because they must forecast the changes in reimbursement for capital expenditures. Without environmental scanning, hospitals will not be able to integrate perceived trends in capital reimbursement with long-range planning for capital expenditures and capital project developments.

## Trustee Education

The board of trustees is responsible for establishing the major mission and aims of a hospital. The precise delegation of authority from the trustees to administrative staff members varies in each hospital, but the trustees generally must approve major strategies and goals that the administrative staff propose, including major capital expenditures for plant and equipment. Responsibility for implementation of broad plans rests with the chief executive officer.

Although the hospital's chief executive officer is responsible for environmental monitoring, the trustees will need to be kept informed about the latest changes in reimbursement systems, prognoses for future changes, and the impact of such changes on the hospital. They will also need to know about possible alternative scenarios if more third party payers adopt prospective reimbursement systems that require greater control over expenditures. Without this information, trustees may not be able to provide the sort of guidance that hospitals need from their board of directors. Thus, executives who wish to help their boards in policy formulation and decision making should provide a periodic, yet steady flow of written information about the changes in hospital reimbursement and should include a brief discussion of the possible implications for the hospital. The educational process should focus primarily on key variables in the hospital environment. In this manner, less time will be spent during board meetings in discussions of specific past, present, and future changes in reimbursement, and more time can be spent on creating, analyzing, and evaluating alternatives.

The extent of trustee education and involvement in the environmental monitoring process is obviously determined by the composition of the board. Since the personalities and professional orientations of hospital board members vary extensively from one hospital to the next, the education requirements may vary. Some board members will need less help than others, but hospital executives need to bring all board members to a similar level of knowledge. The best approach, therefore, is for hospital executives to remain sensitive to their board members and to be prepared to supply information when necessary.

## STRATEGIC PLANS VS. OPERATIONAL PLANS

According to Steiner,[1] it is possible to differentiate among several levels of planning as is shown in this interpretation of his model:

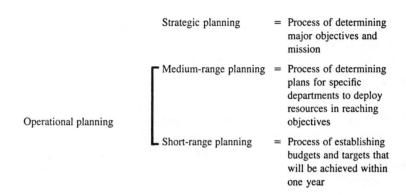

Medium-range planning and short-range planning can be combined as operational planning, which differs from strategic planning, according to Steiner, in its level of conduct, regularity, uncertainty, time frame, and alternatives considered.[2] The top echelons of the hospital carry out strategic planning on a regular basis when uncertainty is high, the alternatives are many, and the time frame covers years. Department level managers carry out operational planning on a regular basis when uncertainty is low, the alternatives are generally more specific and fewer in number, and the time frame covers the forthcoming year (or two). Therefore, a strategy involves defining the major objectives to be achieved (with respect to managing DRGs, for example), while operational plans address the specific methods for achieving those objectives.

There are both strategic and operational aspects in planning for prospective payment. On one hand, hospitals must step back and envision their responses for the next three to five years (assuming that prospective payment systems introduced by third party payers will be fairly congruent with Medicare's DRGs). On the other hand, hospitals must develop a specific operational plan that addresses the constraints imposed by prospective payment in the short run. These short-run plans must not interfere with the long-run strategies, however.

## FORMING STRATEGIC PLANS

It is useful to distinguish between short-run and long-run strategic plans.[3] In the case of prospective payment, there must be initial planning for a shorter time frame (one to two years) that defines specifically how the hospital will manage prospective payment until the long-run strategic plans are operationally applicable. Short-run strategic planning, which sets a basis for specific operational plans, should not commit the hospital to a highly constrained set of expectations.

## Short-Run Strategic Plans

DRG-oriented plans are evolutionary. Plans will change as hospitals learn about the use of DRGs and more fully comprehend their effects on operating policies. The adaptation of a hospital's strategic plans is a long-run process rather than a single event. This view of change is very important because of the magnitude of the change that will accompany DRG-based reimbursement for most hospitals.

Initially, hospital executives must turn their attention to critical short-run problem areas. It will be infeasible for most hospitals to address the 467 DRGs at a single point in time because they lack sufficient administrative resources or they lack an information system that provides quality information for decision making. In short-run planning, executives must prioritize DRGs.

### *Prioritizing*

Hospital executives must identify which DRGs are associated with excessive costs and which generate the bulk of hospital revenue. Once these groups have been identified, the executives can begin to plan solutions which address the reasons for excessive costs in certain case mix categories. Simultaneously, the DRGs that produce excess revenue over costs should be evaluated. If they can ascertain what factors have contributed to the favorable balance, the executives may develop effective management plans for cost control that can be implemented in DRGs without such a favorable balance. This does not mean that simply because a hospital's experience in any one diagnostic category is favorable (i.e., costs are below the level of reimbursement), that the category can be forgotten in the planning process. Patients and their treatment by physicians can differ from one year to the next. What may not be a problem today for a set of diagnostic categories may surface as a problem tomorrow. However, for short-run planning, it is not possible to address every one of the 467 categories.

This suggestion for prioritizing DRGs implicitly incorporates the Pareto Principle,[4] which suggests that 20 percent of all endeavor results in 80 percent of all results. This principle can easily be applied to short-run management and planning strategies for DRGs. Executives focus on the 20 percent of all DRGs that affect 80 percent of excessive costs and 80 percent of surplus revenues.

By means of prioritization, hospital executives can work more efficiently in the short run, allocating their scarce resources—particularly time—to the DRGs with the highest payoff (i.e., added revenue) or the highest potential for payoff (i.e., reduced costs). In addition, prioritization ensures that executives give some attention to traditional decisions and plans, which are not simply going to disappear from management agendas.

In determining which DRGs should receive a high priority, hospital executives must identify the cost per case (and the level of variance) for each DRG. It may be convenient to use ratios (cost per case divided by revenue per case) where

1. those DRGs with a ratio equal to 1 represent breakeven

2. those DRGs with a ratio less than 1 represent favorable inflows

3. those DRGs with a ratio greater than 1 represent excessive costs for services provided

The best strategy for maintaining financial solvency may be to minimize the number of DRGs (weighted by the number of cases per year—case mix) that provide a negative return.

At this point, most hospitals have not adequately defined their product and do not know what it costs to deliver it.[5] Among the first things hospitals must do is to merge two information systems, parallel billing and medical records. The key concept is variable cost change. It will be necessary to monitor length of stay, admissions, amount of care required, medical/surgical case mix, utilization of ancillary services, outpatient utilization, and general physician practice patterns.

One inevitable result of prospective payment is a move toward realistic cost accounting.[6] Hospitals need a cost accounting system that indicates how much each piece of the production process costs. If a hospital does not know how much it costs to provide a particular service, it cannot decide what the charge should be and which services are profitable. Although it took many years to refine and apply cost accounting in the business sector, hospitals must incorporate it very quickly. Most hospitals will start the process in major departments and services, and only gradually involve the entire institution.

The DRGs with ratios greater than 1 must be ranked according to the average number of cases treated in the hospital per year. A good base line for this average might be the number of cases per diagnosis over the last three to five years. In this manner, hospital executives can ascertain not only which DRGs are generating excessive costs, but also which DRGs are important to the caseload of the hospital.

## Plan Development

Once the DRGs or clinical performance areas that generate more costs than revenues have been identified, it is possible to formulate specific operational plans for reversing the deficit. Obviously, the precise components of the plans depend on the DRG and the reasons that costs are higher than revenues.

Executives must investigate cause and effect among the variables in the clinical area:

- Is physician productivity at a low level because the number of trained ancillary staff members is insufficient?
- Are 20 percent of the clinical staff in a department generating excessive costs?
- Are medical and nonmedical staff aware of the excessive costs they are generating?
- Are equipment malfunctions reducing staff productivity?
- Are supply costs rising so much that a new supplier(s) should be contacted?

These and many other questions should be assessed in order to develop a precise operating plan to resolve problems.

Alternately, a hospital may decide to discontinue certain services. Although there are serious ethical and legal problems with this strategy, the hospital may encourage medical staff members to use discretion when referring or accepting patients for treatment. In this fashion, a hospital can prioritize its services. Executives may discover that new policies must be formulated, however, since some services traditionally offered in the hospital are now omitted.

## Long-Run Strategic Plans

Although prioritizing high-cost DRGs will identify clinical and support service areas with excessive costs, a long-run plan must be formulated for reducing costs. Action can move from the conceptual to the practical and the specific.

### Cost Containment Plans

Because of hospitals' failure to control costs, for whatever reasons, third party payers are beginning to adopt prospective reimbursement as one method to achieve a better measure of cost control. This action does not develop the needed cost containment methods, however; it only increases hospitals' motivation to create the controls. At least three areas appear to have merit for planning long-run cost containment programs under DRGs:

1. operations management (i.e., inventory control and patient scheduling)
2. staffing
3. program evaluation

Operations management has always been important for promoting the efficient use of resources in hospitals, but it has sometimes been disregarded when there have been no incentives to pursue greater efficiency. DRG-based reimbursement places a higher premium on the use of resources in all service areas. Control over supply orders and inventory maintenance must become tighter; adequate supplies and buffer amounts must be available for services, but the costs of carrying excessive inventories preclude the slack relied on in the past. Purchases should be integrated within a comprehensive plan. Group purchasing arrangements should form an integral part of this cost control strategy.

Patient scheduling is another operations management area that should be evaluated by administrators who are interested in holding down costs. The focus should be on reducing excess beds while maximizing utilization. Long-run plans that define patient scheduling should support the DRGs that are most consistent with a hospital's service component. Cost containment can best be aided by refining internal operations and maximizing occupancy.

Plans for personnel staffing will assume renewed importance for hospitals that have been overstaffed. Personnel costs per case are excessively high for DRGs that are underutilized or for which the reimbursement rate is so low that certain diagnostic services cannot be provided. There will not be enough cases over the year to reach a point of efficiency. Staff positions will require greater justification under DRG-based reimbursement than in the past.

The cost effectiveness of hospital programs must be evaluated to ensure that a good return is being received for the invested resources. Toleration of both the fixed and the variable costs that accompany any program will be reduced under DRG-based reimbursement; there will be less slack in the total budget, and not every program can be funded. As a result, program directors should be expected to justify their expenditures on capital (e.g., equipment) and noncapital investments. Unless the program directors can present specific plans to maintain or increase cost-effectiveness, hospital executives should consider reducing or eliminating programs that use more resources than they return in revenues. This is an important concept of long-run planning since capital-intensive programs (e.g., those that require substantial investments in technological equipment) may be difficult to justify in terms of caseload as a result of DRGs.

*Medical Staff Plans*

DRG-based reimbursement requires hospital executives to work more closely with their medical staff members. Planning must include the development of mechanisms for cooperation between the administration and medical staff. In conjunction with the medical staff, the administrative staff must improve the structure and process of utilization review. The care of any patient whose length of stay exceeds the average length of stay will negatively affect the hospital's revenue, for example. Thus, utilization review must be upgraded in its efficiency and quality to convey to medical staff the importance of avoiding inappropriate and unnecessary utilization. Under DRG-based reimbursement, the incentive for physicians to control utilization is given to them indirectly through the hospital.

Policies should also be developed in conjunction with the medical staff to discourage the use of supplemental ancillary services that have a negative or low return. The hospital executive must provide information from which the medical staff can decide how to change behavior vis-à-vis ancillary services. These policies can be reinforced either through incentive systems or review of medical staff privileges. Physicians may initially fight these implied controls, but they will also discover that the financially sound hospitals have the most promising professional opportunities.

In the planning and policy-setting process, executives should take into account the need for support services that enable physicians to set meaningful and cost-effective goals. Because prospective reimbursement encourages a decreased length of stay, discharge planning programs must be upgraded to reduce the malpractice risk (to physicians and hospital); to provide the best alternative for patients who need extended care, yet are able to leave the hospital; and to improve the hospital's ability to provide truly appropriate care. Thus, the planning process also involves revising plans for support staff.

*Ancillary Staff Plans*

Most hospital executives clearly understand the importance of working with the medical staff to monitor the medical care process under DRGs, but many overlook the valuable role that the ancillary staff members can play and fail to incorporate these staff members in their plans. Executives must remember, however, that they have a significant degree of control over ancillary staff, which increases their ability to achieve overall cost control, to implement procedural changes, and to visualize cause-and-effect changes. These are essential ingredients of any long-run planning for DRG-based reimbursement.

Although the planned incorporation of ancillary staff into a hospital's cost containment effort usually begins as a policy of limited rewards for good suggestions or additional in-service education on the impact of DRGs on their departments, the most effective plan for control involves the creation and *use* of departmental budgets. Until department heads and supervisors are rewarded or penalized for the performance of their departments, cost control will remain elusive. Hospital executives must instill the notion of merit pay for performance; otherwise, they should expect little beyond mediocre results.

*Information System Plans*

For most hospitals, developing and refining the information system must be given a high priority in long-run planning. The need for accurate and timely information on cost per diagnosis, case mix, and average length of stay (for example) is immediate under DRG-based reimbursement. Unless hospitals are able to identify areas of cost overruns accurately and quickly, it is unlikely that they will be able to formulate the necessary changes in their delivery of services. Thus, they will be unable to hold down costs while maximizing revenues.

Essentially, good information makes it possible to identify cost deviances. Once these areas of deviance have been spotted, medical and administrative staff can consider various trade-offs in those areas. They are better prepared to decide among eliminating a service area, investing more resources (e.g., capital investment in equipment that increases the productivity of personnel) in that area, or making no changes for the moment.

For most hospitals, the implementation of DRG-based reimbursement has provided ample incentive to fine-tune information systems in order to manage problem areas (i.e., those in which costs are greater than revenue). Information systems must be developed in a methodical and timely manner; they should be based on a model that will allow for changes as DRGs evolve. Hospital executives should avoid creating an information system so inflexible that it must be reconstructed every time a new health policy is introduced.

## FORMING OPERATIONAL PLANS

The precise tactics—deployment of resources—for implementing strategic plans depend on the nature and goals of the plans themselves. All hospitals have at least one common goal—cost control. There are a number of tactics that hospitals can use in controlling costs and enhancing revenue.

### Reduction/Elimination of Services

Programs with low cost-effectiveness must be carefully assessed with an eye toward reducing or eliminating them. Many of these programs (e.g., social services, collaborative teaching or educational associations, and community education) were originally designed to support patients and to make them appreciate the hospital. Although such programs have been viewed as essential in the past, they may now represent an increasingly untenable cost burden under the revenue restrictions of prospective payment. Patients may want the services offered in these programs, but hospitals can no longer subsidize non–revenue-producing services and programs.

Prospective reimbursement may produce a return to basic hospital services as one method of cost control. This approach entails the elimination of nonmedical services or the expansion of cost sharing by patients in supporting these services. The focus is on streamlining hospital programs and providing medical care without frills. Hospitals and patients alike may be less pleased with these austerity programs, but the rate of national expenditures on health care services suggests that a more restrained concept of medical care may be appropriate.

As a variation on the reduction or elimination of services, hospitals may offer amenity packages that patients can purchase. The entire episode of care may be upgraded in terms of support services if the patient is willing to pay for nonreimbursable support services. The hospital may wish to subsidize the support services to keep the co-payment at a level tolerable to the patient. Yet, this co-payment would encourage patients to use only those services in which they are most interested.

## Subcontracts for Services

Some hospitals provide services through subcontractors. A hospital must, again, carefully assess its options when considering the use of subcontractors. If a small hospital in which the laundry has never attained the desired level of efficiency and productivity faces expenditures for new laundry equipment, for example, the hospital may contemplate subcontracting services. Perhaps the food service has been a source of constant cost or quality problems; with the advent of prospective reimbursement, a hospital may decide to subcontract food services, thereby eliminating substantial fixed and variable costs (although also eliminating flexibility and increasing risk because of the hospital's dependence on an agency outside its control).

Subcontracts need not be limited to support services, but can also include direct medical care. The spiraling cost of equipment may cause a hospital to subcontract for certain radiology or laboratory services. Even though these areas have always been lucrative hospital services in the past, prospective payment establishes a new environment that requires a fresh view of all hospital services. New combinations of services may be more appropriate over the long run, depending on the goal of the hospital.

## Multi-Institutional Alliances

One method of cost containment that has been advocated in the health care literature is a multi-institutional alliance.[7-9] In such alliances, hospitals may either share services/facilities or participate in group purchasing plans that allow them to take advantage of economies of scale to drive down costs for the individual hospital. The magnitude of the cost savings can vary with the service or purchase, but the value of the group association is its ability to obtain consistent cost reductions on a multitude of items.

Although a hospital may join a multi-institutional group as part of its cost containment plan, it is important to recognize that something will be sacrificed in the process. Many health care facilities discover that they must sacrifice choice and quality (control) when they join a group plan. This sort of trade-off may not be consistent with other plans that the hospital deems important. Such a conflict between cost and quality appears to be inevitable in the health care field; hospitals must maximize both to the extent that each constrains the other.

Hospitals in a multi-institutional alliance may also find that they have abdicated their autonomy. Cook, Shortell, Conrad, and Morrisey argued, however, that hospitals will be forced into multi-institutional alliances in order to acquire a degree of control—or autonomy from—the external regulatory environment.[10] Since prospective reimbursement can easily be viewed as quasi-regulation, this theory, if valid, will be evident in a higher number of multi-institutional groups in the hospital field. These groups may increase their autonomy from regulatory control by means of collective bargaining with regulatory agencies. Of course, hospitals will lose some autonomy as they give up freedom of choice (in purchases) when they join the multi-institutional alliance.

### Outpatient Care

Hospitals may need to perform a greater number of medical procedures on an outpatient basis, because the *proportional* benefits of revenue over costs are greater for outpatient care than for inpatient care. The implementation of prospective payment systems will encourage patients and hospitals to avoid inpatient care, if possible. In addition, patients who are admitted will be more rapidly discharged and referred to day care facilities. As the average length of stay decreases, the amount of profit will increase per case. Yet some mechanism must be developed to cope with the marginal cases that can be referred home, but require some minimal monitoring or additional recuperative services. The possibilities here are virtually unlimited for the creative hospital and medical staff.

Physicians can be encouraged to conduct more extensive preadmission testing. The more diagnostic tests that are undertaken on an outpatient basis and, hence, reimbursed under retrospective payment, the greater the revenue per case once patients are admitted; this approach may provide substantial cost savings to the hospital once the patient is admitted. This approach requires not only a revision in medical care patterns, but also significant adjustments in hospitals' diagnostic equipment and outpatient departments.

## TOWARD COST CONTROL PLANS

The ability of hospitals to plan for cost control hinges on their ability to implement careful planning strategies. The elimination or reduction of services, outpatient care, use of subcontractors for services, and multi-institutional alliances are not necessarily new ideas, but they are significant cost control strategies that may require more consideration in the future. Clearly, the best planning for prospective reimbursement will incorporate a fresh perspective on more traditional and even contemporary plans for cost control. With relatively slight modifications in these plans, it may be possible to create entirely new programs that not only help hospitals provide better care, but also result in substantially lower costs for the health care system.

---

## NOTES

1. George A. Steiner, *Strategic Planning* (New York: Free Press, 1979), 4.

2. George A. Steiner, *Top Management Planning* (London: Macmillan, 1969).

3. Peter Lorange and Richard F. Vancil, *Strategic Planning Systems* (Englewood Cliffs, N.J.: Prentice-Hall, 1977).

4. Howard L. Smith and Richard A. Reid, "Short and Long Run Management Strategies for DRGs," *Hospital Topics* 62(1984): 4–40.

5. Emily Friedman, "Getting to Know Us: Hospitals May Finally Learn about True Cost and Pricing," *Hospitals* 57(March 16, 1983): 74–82.

6. "Strategies for Change," *Hospitals* 57 (July 1, 1983): 58–63.

7. Bernard Friedman, William Pierskalla, and Tryfon Beazoglow, "Sharing Arrangements in the Non-profit Hospital Industry," *Health Services Research* 14 (Summer 1979): 150–159.

8. Myron D. Fottler, John R. Schermerhorn, and John Wong, "Multi-Institutional Arrangements in Health Care: Some Marketing Implications," *Journal of Health Care Marketing* 1 (Winter 1981):45–58.

9. Myron D. Fottler, John R. Schermerhorn, John Wong, and William Money, "Multi-Institutional Arrangements in Health Care," *Academy of Management Review* 7 (January 1982): 67–79.

10. Karen Cook, Stephen M. Shortell, Douglas A. Conrad, and Michael A. Morrisey, "A Theory of Organizational Response to Regulation: The Case of Hospitals," *Academy of Management Review* 8 (April 1983): 193–205.

# Chapter 4

# Strategic Factors: Identifying Services and Markets

Although cost containment might be viewed as the main purpose of prospective payment systems, hospital executives must be alert to the broader ramifications of changes in the method of reimbursement. Even hospitals that develop strategic plans centered around cost containment may overlook other factors that are vital to the successful management of prospective payment and DRGs.

After the selection of cost containment strategies, perhaps the biggest decision confronting hospitals is the selection of services and markets to be served over the long run.

## DEVELOPMENT OF A VISION

Strategic planning requires an explicit focus on a hospital's external environment, market, internal operations, and competitive advantage. All these should be analyzed *prior* to actual goal setting. Hospital executives should scan expected changes in the health care environment in order to identify the hospital's particular opportunities and constraints. The scanning process usually involves a group of five to ten decision makers from the hospital executive staff and key board members. These individuals discuss anticipated changes in an open forum and attempt to determine the economic, legal/political, international, technological, social/demographic, and competitive opportunities and constraints facing the hospital.

In assessing changes in the market for health care services, the scanning group may develop a profile of the patients presently served by the hospital and compare it to a similar patient profile of the past and the anticipated profile of the future. Since the hospital serves more than one group (e.g., patients and physicians), several profiles must be developed. In order to obtain this information, the group may need to review historical data, complete a patient or physician survey, engage a market research firm, read materials on their service area, review census data, or use a panel of patients and/or physicians for in-depth questioning. The strategic planning group should examine the profiles from at least four perspectives:

1. demographics (age, sex, location, income level)
2. motivation/needs (security, prestige, status, values)
3. social/behavioral factors (purchase patterns, sophistication)
4. service expectations

In most hospitals, demographic changes and social/behavioral changes are weighted most heavily.

A good way for the planning group to assess the internal strengths and weaknesses of the hospital is to ask themselves two questions about the entire hospital and about their particular division: (1) What is it we do really well? and (2) What is it we have problems with? Typically, strengths or weaknesses are identified in such areas as personnel, physician facilities, equipment, location, cash and other assets, reputation, special products/services/markets, and market position.

On the basis of the data generated, the group can begin to determine the competitive advantage(s) of the particular hospital. A clear image of what makes the hospital stand out and what the hospital does well is necessary in order to set more specific goals and objectives.

At this point, the group is ready to write goals and objectives. These should reflect major areas of organizational effort (e.g., new services, growth in outpatient care, revenue increases, markct penetration, or personnel changes), should be specific and measurable, and should include a date by which the goal or objective is to be achieved. For example, the goal might be to increase local market penetration in pediatric services from 16 percent in 1984 to 25 percent by 1987. Any specific objective should reflect the major strengths of the organization, take advantage of the environmental opportunities, and avoid or minimize external constraints. One individual should be held accountable for the achievement of each objective.

Once the strategic goals have been determined, implementation must be considered. The major steps or activities required to reach a strategic objective must be identified, and who will do what, when, and the method by which progress will be tracked or measured must be specified.

The assessment of the major strengths and weaknesses of the hospital, the creation of a vision of mission, and the planning for eventual implementation are the most important decisions to be made by hospital leadership. This vision not only provides a hospital staff with a concept of common purpose, but also helps to differentiate one hospital from another. Hospitals need to be recognized for distinction in terms of either goals or the provision of certain services. A hospital may become known for its broad array of birthing packages, for example, or for its exceptional pediatric surgery program. Another hospital may emphasize its combination of outpatient and inpatient geriatric services.

Hospitals cannot allow the implementation of prospective reimbursement to channel their strategic plans for services and markets into mediocrity. A hospital may not have the resources to be the best in several service areas, but it can pursue a vision of excellence for certain areas. Although plans and specific tactics for implementation must be made and revised as the hospital progresses toward its goal(s), the vision should not be put aside simply because prospective payment creates a more difficult environment. Without a firm commitment from the top echelons of the trustees, administration, and medical staff, however, the hospital may never attain distinction for a given component of services or markets.

## MARKET ASSESSMENT UNDER DRGs

Creating a vision to guide hospitals under prospective reimbursement is very different from creating a vision to guide them under retrospective reimbursement. Hospitals had greater slack in their budgets under retrospective payment and, hence, were able to pursue many programs. Although this same attitude can prevail under prospective payment—with very careful planning—the set of constraints is expanded. Prospective payment encourages more conservatism, less expansion, and greater attention to current operations. Alternatives are now more limited. Less experimentation is likely, since the current capacity and capabilities of hospitals are known and measurable. New programs have a higher risk because the costs and revenues associated with them are not known, not easily projected, and not conducive to immediate return on investment.

The difference between market planning by hospitals under retrospective reimbursement and that under prospective reimbursement illustrates the essence of the hospital executive's dilemma (Figure 4–1). No longer can growth occur whenever and wherever the hospital desires. Now the constraints of reimbursement begin to take effect, and they must be actively incorporated in the decision-making and planning process. Optimism can prevail, however, because external regulation and reimbursement have not totally eliminated the capacity for executives and trustees to manage their facilities as they wish.[1,2]

### Market Planning under Retrospective Reimbursement

The general process of market planning under retrospective reimbursement begins with the analysis of existing services and patient care, with an emphasis on the strengths and weaknesses of the hospital in providing those services. Numerous specific criteria may be used in this assessment:

**Figure 4–1** Market Planning under Retrospective and Prospective Reimbursement

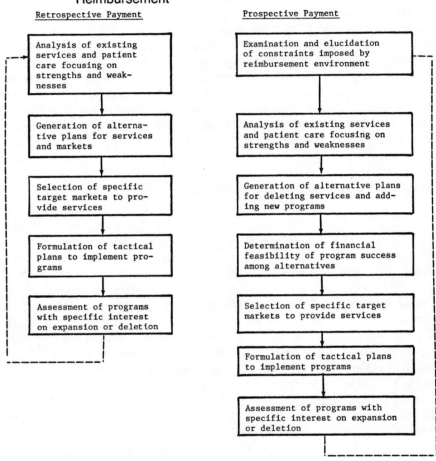

- cost per unit of service
- quality of services delivered
- integration of the services within an overall plan for services
- financial return on the services from an inpatient view
- financial return from associated outpatient services
- ability to expand the services in the future

After existing patient care services and markets have been analyzed, the hospital can proceed to generate plans for alternative services and markets. Under retrospective reimbursement, the opportunities are almost as wide as the imagination of the hospital staff and the availability of resources. The ability to pass on costs made it possible to give programs more time to develop before they were deemed failures.

Following the generation of alternative plans for services and markets, a specific target market must be selected. Under retrospective reimbursement, this decision process requires tough-minded analysis of underlying premises, continual reference to the overall mission of the hospital, and consideration of the compatibility of the proposed alternative with the existing services. The hospital must avoid a patchwork quilt of programs that are difficult to integrate, are difficult to manage, are difficult for patients to identify, and fail to enhance the hospital's reputation as a leader. Under retrospective payment, this sort of analysis is more easily postponed, since there is no real financial penalty for cost-ineffective clinical services. Even high-risk projects are feasible under retrospective payment.

Retrospective reimbursement also affects the tactical plans for implementation of the clinical programs selected. Cost control is less urgent; there is a longer time frame for implementation planning in which revenues can be built up. Thus, a radiologist who proposes that the hospital replace a computerized axial tomography (CAT) scanner with a Nuclear Magnetic Imager (NMI) may worry less about justifying the long-run payoff of the equipment to the board of trustees. Retrospective payment buffers the implementation phase, providing a measure of slack that does not necessarily encourage rigorous analysis.

Finally, retrospective reimbursement provides little incentive for hospital executives to review prior decisions. Since costs are not critical (because of direct reimbursement), virtually any clinical program can prove successful. As a result, hospital executives may assume that every decision previously made is a good decision and may not see the need to reevaluate programs. This reluctance to review prior decisions is detrimental to the performance of any hospital. Even with the shift to more lean and more efficient hospitals in the last decade, the administrative reluctance to reevaluate that which hospitals are producing—services, return on equity, and satisfaction of consumers—has remained.

## Market Planning under Prospective Reimbursement

Under prospective reimbursement, hospitals must first conduct an in-depth analysis of the constraints imposed by the reimbursement environment,[3] particularly as they affect the retention of services, the deletion of services, and the possible expansion of services. The focus is on current clinical and support services, the need for them, the financial return on them, and the possibilities for deleting or expanding them. Secondary consideration is given to services not yet offered by the hospital. Because this analysis takes place within the context of possible financial restraint, the attitude toward planning is one of greater conservatism and caution.

The analysis of hospital strengths and weaknesses is tempered by an increasingly important financial criterion under prospective reimbursement. Hospital executives must determine whether a clinical department is a liability or an asset under prospective payment; they must determine whether it produces positive cash flows or, at a minimum, breaks even while allowing another clinical unit to produce net income. Existing services must be considered for revision or deletion. Investment of the valuable resources that they consume could provide a higher return if invested in other services. For every clinical program that is not carrying its weight, the hospital must respond with a similar program that compensates for negative income flows.

The generation of new program alternatives under prospective reimbursement is only superficially similar to that under retrospective reimbursement. Under prospective payment, opportunities to act in an entrepreneurial manner are much more limited, because the time frame for financial solvency is much shorter. Entrepreneurial tendencies must be checked by a criterion of return on investment. The set of alternatives that can be generated is smaller, since hospital executives must focus on financial feasibility. They must also ascertain the secondary costs and benefits of these progams. In contrast, under retrospective payment, programs have been evaluated on cost-effectiveness, not revenue-generating capacity, at both the primary and secondary levels.

After financial feasibility has been determined, market planning under prospective reimbursement proceeds as it does under retrospective reimbursement. Fewer new programs will have been selected and more detailed marketing efforts will accompany the new programs, however. Above all, hospitals cannot afford to initiate a succession of failures. Thus, more clinical, administrative, and marketing resources must be invested in making certain that programs succeed.

The formulation of tactical plans to implement programs also proceeds with greater caution under prospective payment. Attention must be directed to cost projections and anticipated net revenues. The fact that the reimbursement rate is known helps hospital executives in tactical planning. They can generate alternative scenarios for each program in terms of patient use and associated costs.

Finally, the market planning process ends with the assessment of the program expansion or deletion. Under prospective payment, each new program must be considered a trial. In order to be retained, a new program must be profitable. Hospitals cannot afford now or in the future to support an excessive number of unprofitable programs. There will always be programs that generate more costs than revenues under prospective payment, but the hospital must minimize this number.

The deletion of programs that do not produce the intended results does not imply that hospital executives have performed poorly. External regulation, personnel resources, patient demographics, patient preferences, and medical staff change. Such changes are inevitable and healthy for all organizations. Under the right conditions, even the most successful program may be subject to revision or deletion.

## DRG INCENTIVES FOR SERVICE SPECIALIZATION

The implementation of prospective payment systems based on diagnosis-related groups (DRGs) creates a situation in which there is less flexibility for expansion and more need for specialization. Such a system promotes greater efficiency within the hospital by directing attention to ongoing efforts rather than expansion.

Within each DRG for which it provides services, the hospital must contain costs under a fixed rate in order to receive a return of revenue and remain financially viable. As a result, the financial benefit of providing services for those DRGs under which the hospital has net income is an incentive for the hospital to specialize in those DRGs.

Once the profitable DRGs have been identified, the hospital has several choices. It is difficult to eliminate all services for which costs exceed revenues in most general service hospitals, because services overlap. Therefore, it may be feasible to discontinue heart transplants within the hospital, but not bypass surgery. It may be appropriate to forego kidney transplants  but not the treatment of kidney disease. Furthermore, kidney dialysis may not be offered, even though general kidney and urinary tract surgery is offered.

## SPECIALIZATION STRATEGIES

The DRG rate, the resources available to the hospital, the treatment patterns, and the vision that the hospital has for its services determine the strategy of specialization. The DRG rate establishes a standard against which hospitals can judge their performance and on which they can base specialization plans.

### General Specialization

A hospital may decide to continue providing a complement of general services rather than to rely on orthopedics, oncology, nephrology, or another clinical department. This strategy begins with a longitudinal analysis of the hospital's performance in all DRGs in order to ascertain which DRGs consistently generate revenue that exceeds costs and which do not.

Once the most costly DRGs have been identified, hospital executives must assess the likelihood that cost control measures will be effective. Some hospitals will find that they can no longer afford to provide some of the services that they have provided in the past. This break with tradition may create some conflict with the medical staff, and some staff members may transfer to hospitals that concentrate on their specialization. Although not desirable, this course of events is probably inevitable unless the medical staff is willing to participate in the compromises necessary to keep their hospitals financially solvent.

If there are no feasible plans for holding down costs for a particular DRG, deletion of that DRG from the list of hospital services must be considered. Quality assurance programs should be taken into account in this determination. A correlation between high cost and high risk (i.e., malpractice) in a DRG makes that DRG a candidate for termination. Naturally, the medical staff, administration, and board of trustees should participate fully in the decision to terminate any DRG-based services. The administrative staff must carefully document all assertions that providing services for a given DRG is too costly. In the end, compromise will probably lead to a satisfactory resolution. Plans may then be made for a reassessment of all marginal DRG deletions and retentions one year after the decision-making process has concluded.

After the DRG service component has been determined for the general specialization strategy, the hospital must formulate tactical plans to implement an organizationwide cost containment program. The purpose of the cost control program is to ensure that the selected DRGs do not result in cost overruns. Since the hospital cannot predict the rate of increase (i.e., inflation) in future DRG rates, it must control that which is under its purview—its internal costs and the variables associated with those costs.

## Specific Specialization

Like general specialization, specific specialization requires an assessment of all DRGs to determine where costs exceed revenues. Using data on costs, revenues, average length of stay, and related decision variables, the medical staff, hospital administration, and board of trustees must determine which areas of specialty medical care are the distinguishing capabilities of the hospital. Once these clusters of DRGs have been identified and analyzed, further plans about the medical care that the hospital will provide, such as the best use of ancillary personnel, equipment, and facilities, can be formulated.

Specialization may be a radical change in a hospital's traditional method of operation. Even though the most lucrative DRGs comprise the heart of the hospital's service component, with every risk comes the possibility of failure. Thus, estimates and changes should probably be conservative. Furthermore, it is unlikely that hospitals will be able to reduce the number of their lucrative DRGs drastically. At least for the first four years of the Medicare payment system, there is considerable latitude in rate determination, which will minimize the tendency of hospitals and medical staffs to specialize.

A hospital that has decided to concentrate on its most lucrative DRGs is not exempt from planning for cost control. A long-run perspective is needed in order to recognize the dangers of unfavorable DRG rates and to compensate for them in advance. Once a hospital's costs exceed its level of reimbursement, it has a poor prognosis for the future. Hence, administrators must instill a greater awareness of the need for cost control among staff members; this is most easily done when the threat is low and the cost control orientation can be phased in gradually.

## General vs. Specific Specialization

The general specialization strategy is a management approach that relies on efficiency (Figure 4–2). It emphasizes reductions in costs to attain its goals. In contrast, the specific specialization strategy promotes marketing with less emphasis on operational efficiency; it is based on the premise that a hospital should lead from its best position, attracting patients to its most lucrative DRGs. Cost containment or efficiency may receive less emphasis under this strategy because the hospital has greater revenue (per unit) initially.

These strategies also differ in the degree of specialization. The general strategy is obviously low in specialization and maintains the overall framework of general inpatient care. The specific specialization strategy, by definition, involves extreme specialization, with other services retained merely as support for the areas of specialization.

The general specialization strategy involves relatively little risk to the hospital, because it simply discontinues services for costly DRGs. This may have been the goal of hospital administrators for some time, but the implementation of DRG-based reimbursement has only now supplied an incentive to achieve the goal. Because relatively few services have been terminated, the hospital with a general strategy is in a position to react favorably to future DRG rate changes; after all, the favorable DRG rate of today may be the unfavorable rate of tomorrow. Hospitals that follow the specific specialization strategy accept the risk of DRG rate changes in the belief that their efficiency in performing a limited number of services will maximize their income, even if the DRG rates change.

The general specialization strategy offers a low return from service, because the hospital continues to provide services for DRGs that are unprofitable, as well as for those that are profitable. The results will probably balance each other, but the return to the hospital will be low. Under the specific specialization strategy, revenue can be maximized and a high return achieved. Careful safeguards must be built into the plan for specialization, however; the return may diminish, for example, if cost containment is overlooked or if the externally set rates fluctuate widely over time. Most likely it will be this external variability that will cause many hospitals to retain the general specialization model. Hospitals that follow the

**Figure 4–2** Strategies for DRG Specialization

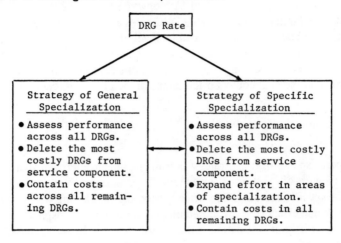

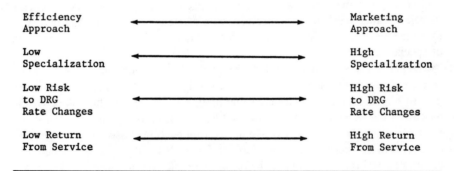

specific specialization model must be closely attuned to relative changes in DRG rates and willing to make modifications in the service mix.

## PITFALLS OF HASTY DRG SELECTION

A hospital's hasty selection of DRGs may send it down a path that weakens its long-run competitive position. Although it seems preferable to specialize in the lucrative DRGs, it is necessary to consider whether they are lucrative in actuality, what would happen if all the hospitals in the area concentrated on the same DRGs, and what would happen if all hospitals dropped the same DRGs simultaneously.

Assume that 100 hospitals are able to attain a net income per case for 50 specific DRGs at point $\overline{X}_0$ on the normal curve (Figure 4–3). Assume that the hospitals ($n = 50$) that exceed the mean score make a profit, while those below the mean score ($n = 50$) lose money. Those 50 facilities that are losing money opt to concentrate on other DRGs. Therefore, in Year 1 of the specialization strategy, the specializers discover that the normal curve and mean score have moved to the right of $\overline{X}_1$. With variability in service from one year to the next, some are now actually losing money on the DRGs on which they have decided to concentrate.

Meanwhile, the regional reimbursement agency (e.g., Medicare) observes this trend and responds by lowering the DRG rate, such that net income per case drops to point $\overline{X}_2$ (or perhaps even $\overline{X}_0$). Because of this reduction in the DRG rate, costs exceed revenues in more specialist hospitals. The rate will continue to fluctuate in accordance with the reimbursement agency's perception of a statistically acceptable rate of return. That rate (e.g., $\overline{X}_2$) may be higher than initially established by the agency (e.g., $\overline{X}_0$). With only the most efficient hospitals now concentrating on the DRGs, however, the rate is likely to be driven down because the high cost facilities have dropped out of the market. Specialization can then have undesired effects.

In a hasty selection of DRGs, hospital executives may also overlook the inadequacies of the hospital's information system. Many artifacts in information systems can preclude a correct interpretation of cause and effect. Therefore, hospital executives must proceed with the utmost caution when they select DRGs in which to specialize. They must determine, for example, whether any unusual operating advantages (e.g., investment in equipment that can be realized for two to three years before heavy reinvestment is needed again) have resulted in the favorable DRG or whether the DRG in question is benefiting from another area where the fixed costs are already covered.

In selecting DRGs from among the 467, hospital executives may fail to take into account the realities of hospitals and physician behavior. The fact that many DRGs use the same resources (e.g., surgical equipment, therapeutic equipment, and nursing staff time) cannot be denied. Separating such DRGs would eliminate the economies of scale that a hospital obtains from pooling its resources in medical care. Furthermore, physicians may refrain from some highly specialized treatments, but they will continue to provide a broad range of services. They must. Physicians do not always know how treatment will progress or what supplemental diagnoses are possible if the patient undergoes surgery. Physicians must be prepared to react to various patient needs; hospitals cannot discourage them from providing general treatment—only very specialized and surgically intensive care.

## TYPICAL HOSPITAL DRG CONCENTRATION

Despite the preceding discussions on how hospitals can manage their DRGs to select only the most lucrative areas, it is still important to recognize that the

**Figure 4–3** Statistical Perturbations Resulting from DRG Selection

Average net revenue
per case for 100
hospitals on 50
specific
DRGs

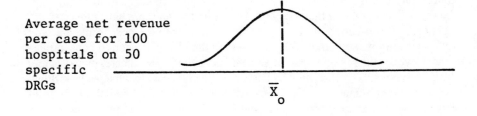

$\overline{X}_o$

Average net revenue per
case for 50 hospitals
which now specialize
on the 50 specific
DRGs--
Year 1

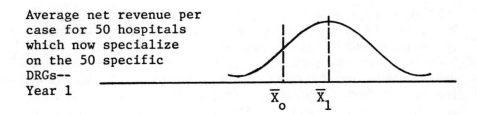

$\overline{X}_o$    $\overline{X}_1$

Average net revenue per
case for 50 hospitals
which specialize on
the 50 specific
DRGs--
Year 2

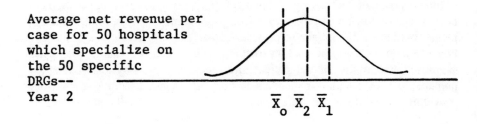

$\overline{X}_o$  $\overline{X}_2$  $\overline{X}_1$

general hospital's concentration on service areas will not drastically change. The foregoing exploration of market planning has progressed from the viewpoint that hospitals want to move beyond reaction toward proactive management of prospective payment. Strategically, this shift in emphasis will occur where hospital executives are cognizant of the implications of DRGs. But, the average hospital will probably not adopt radical specialization. What then is the portrait of the typical hospital's DRG concentration?'

The constraints over most hospitals will prevent them from selecting only lucrative DRGs as their specialized service areas. Rural hospitals and hospitals that are community centers for acute care will find that they are restricted to the general hospital model in which patients who need specialized surgery, for example, must be referred to regional medical centers.

Rural hospitals, in particular, have a community responsibility that transgresses the normal bounds of DRG management. They must be alert to the problems of excessive referral, yet they must not attempt to be everything to everybody. They must also seek to prevent excessive specialization that would make them a liability rather than an asset to their communities.

The typical hospital's DRG concentration will probably be little different from the existing configuration of services. From a practical point of view, hospital executives will be involved in identifying DRGs for which their hospitals have consistent cost overruns. These outliers will receive the bulk of management attention and may be labeled restricted services in the future operations of the hospital. This depends, of course, on the number of deviant cases (i.e., cases with costs higher than revenues) that the hospital has. For the most part, hospitals may not be able to make radical changes in the complexion of their services. Management control requires the expenditure of resources—notably staff time—to identify and monitor unfavorable DRGs. Then, this system must somehow be adapted to the characteristics and demands of the medical staff, who are often reluctant to change their practice patterns. Top management may discover at this point that the medical staff has effectively coopted their control.

Finally, the typical hospital's DRG portrait will not be substantially modified because specialization may produce diminishing returns in the long run. If a high percentage of hospitals gravitate toward the lucrative DRGs, it may be in a hospital's best interest to remain outside this battle and to concentrate on a more stable DRG component with marginally lower returns. Administrators must monitor the trends in their region before selecting strategic action.

## CHANGING EMPHASIS ON PROGRAM DEVELOPMENT

The hospital as an organization has experienced a significant change in its environment. A high proportion of administrative resources that would normally be focused on program planning and operations management must be allocated to this environmental shift. Therefore, fewer new services and programs will be approved; hospital administrators will be focused on streamlining services to attain cost control. In order to be legitimately considered when hospitals are confronting their biggest cost containment challenge, a new program must demonstrate remarkable profitability, help clinical and ancillary services contain costs, raise employee productivity, or generate a substantial number of new patients.

Sometimes, a new program can be used as a marketing or promotional device. As a hospital gravitates toward extreme specialization, it may use various forms of promotional media to create a public awareness of the hospital's narrowing focus. Patients are then channeled into a specific inpatient route. For example, a hospital-based group practice may develop a geriatric medicine program to serve senior citizens.[4] The outpatient component of the program may operate near the break-even point through referrals for inpatient care. The promotional effort by the hospital-based group practice would not center on the inpatient care (except to underscore the easy referral patterns), but rather on the outpatient program. The key is to seek a return on investment at the program level. Once such supporting programs demonstrate their profitability, they must be matched with overall plans for DRG specialization. It is essential to avoid adding programs that do not support the overall mission of the hospital or its DRG program.

As the pressure for cost control grows, patients may be required to self-fund those extra services and amenities not covered by third party payers. It is possible that they will be asked to cover the difference between a hospital's actual cost and the DRG rate for a given acute care episode. This alternative is an equitable one— it requires patients to pay for the amenities they use. If other hospitals in the community do not institute similar patient fees, however, there is likely to be an adverse marketing reaction.

## MARKETING TO MEDICAL STAFF MEMBERS

The medical staff actually determines the success of DRG management, and hospital executives and boards of trustees are likely to pressure the medical staff to keep costs in line. Habitual abusers will probably lose their staff privileges. Furthermore, physicians who seek to join the medical staff may be required to undergo an intensive scrutinizing process. Medical staff privileges will truly become just that—privileges. This is the best form of marketing to physicians that is available, since perhaps more than any other aspect of motivation, physicians are stimulated by professional challenges. Hospitals must capitalize on this allegiance to professional standards in quality of care and cost control. It is a subtle and inexpensive form of marketing, yet it can produce high returns.

Obviously, control of the medical staff's composition extends to the DRGs that are served. If physicians who would *routinely* provide care in those DRGs for which a low or negative cash flow is possible are not on the staff, it is difficult to achieve a regular level of service to these DRGs. A policy that limits medical care activities in prespecified DRGs without prior approval is considered a marketing strategy because it indicates to physicians that the hospital promotes certain areas of medical care. This strategy begins with a decision of the board of trustees, administration, and medical director on which DRGs require prior approval and how the approval is to be obtained. Those physicians who continue to serve these DRGs will realize that the administration is especially interested in these "special" cases. This implied control may be sufficient to achieve the cost containment objective.

Finally, marketing efforts can be directed to medical staff members through continuing education programs about the problems in DRG management. Physicians must be informed about the constraints that DRGs impose on hospitals and the ramifications of medical decisions in the outcome for reimbursement. A realistic portrait of the new environment must be presented to the physicians with the desires of the hospital clearly specified. It should be emphasized that hospitals (all hospitals) are at a juncture where they need cooperation from all physicians. Continuing education should reinforce the concept that both hospital and physician are affected by DRGs.

## CHARITABLE CASES MARKET SEGMENT

One of the more sensitive areas of DRG management is the issue of charitable care. Under retrospective reimbursement, hospitals were able to pass on their costs for charitable care to third party payers. Among these costs were the costs of care for people who could not pay and for people who would not pay. Thus, the burden of charity (and bad debts) was borne by all third party payers and by patients themselves. Under prospective payment, this type of cost shifting and cost sharing will be more limited, because the third party payers have in effect capped the level of reimbursement. Yet someone must pay for the charity. Obviously, hospitals will continue to pass some of these costs on to consumers. It appears, however, that some major perturbations will result for charity care, because hospitals will have well-defined markets—and charitable care will not be one of those markets.

A dual system of health care may develop in which the services available to charity patients are radically different from those available to regular paying patients. This has been a reality of the health system for decades, but the differences will now be magnified. Hospitals will minimize the services they provide to charity patients, and the quality of those services—that is, ancillary services—may be very different. There will be few amenities, and patients will be forced to invest more time (e.g., waiting for slack periods in the provision of services).

Whether the implementation of DRG-based reimbursement will force some hospitals to concentrate so highly on profitable markets that they must refuse to provide charitable care remains to be seen. There can be little doubt that DRGs will have a substantial negative impact on charitable care. This may be the price that our society must pay in order to contain health costs. It is hoped that these trends will be offset by greater philanthropic efforts by all individuals.

## KURTOSIS AND MARKET PLANNING

The statistical term *kurtosis* defines the degree of flatness or vertical height of a normal (bell-shaped) curve. With a flat normal curve, there is a wide standard deviation from the mean score (Figure 4–4). In DRG terms, a flat curve signifies that hospitals have a wide range of costs for a given DRG rate. A more vertical curve indicates that the hospitals cluster around the DRG rate with little variance from that mean score.

Figure 4–4 shows that the DRG mean score $\overline{X}_1$ is formulated at Year 1 around the regional cost data for all hospitals. Hospitals to the left of $\overline{X}_1$ receive net income. Hospitals to the right of $\overline{X}_1$ are operating at a loss and must contain costs in order to operate profitably. This incentive to bring costs into line with the level of reimbursement affects the kurtosis of the curve, because all hospitals will eventually seek the mean. With the inflationary rise of costs, those hospitals that have enjoyed a profitable position will gravitate toward the mean. Thus, kurtosis will change the shape of the curve.

After a year of costs that are higher than revenues, the hospitals to the right of the $\overline{X}_1$ will achieve cost control. By Year 2, the curve has heightened vertically and lost some of its flatness. The mean score $\overline{X}_2$ may or may not remain the same as $\overline{X}_1$, but the curve will narrow. All hospitals are developing similar cost-revenue profiles by Year 2.

The process is taken one step further in Year 3. Once again, the new mean $\overline{X}_3$ may or may not remain the same as $\overline{X}_1$ or $\overline{X}_2$, but the curve is progressively taller and has lost its flatness. The hospitals continue to seek a common cost profile for the given DRG. Cost containment efforts and market (for the DRG) drop-outs continue to prevent excessive skewing of the curve. In the extrapolation of this process, there will be a very narrow range of costs, because all costs and revenues will have been normalized around the DRG rate.

From a marketing perspective, this scenario is rather alarming. It suggests that concentration on a particular set of DRGs because of their profitability will be detrimental over the long run. These trends have not yet been observed, however. Furthermore, it is not likely that costs can be controlled as completely as this

**Figure 4–4** Problems of Kurtosis of DRG Means

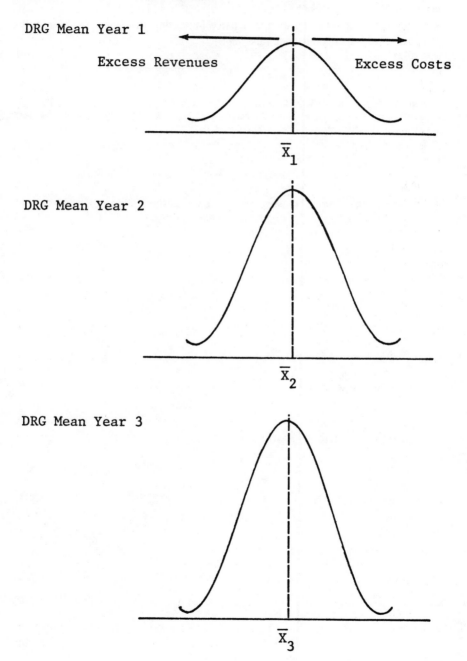

analysis assumes, and the rates themselves may change, depending on unspecified criteria. Thus, it appears that hospital executives should worry less about kurtosis and more about developing comprehensive marketing strategies that build upon the past successes of their hospitals.

---

**NOTES**

1. Karen Cook, Stephen M. Shortell, Douglas A. Conrad, and Michael A. Morrisey, "A Theory of Organizational Response to Regulation: The Case of Hospitals," *Academy of Management Review* 8 (April 1983): 193–205.

2. Howard L. Smith and Stephen M. Mick, "A Theory of Hospital Response to Regulation: A Reply," *Academy of Management Review,* in press.

3. Peter Bruton, "A Reasoned Approach to Hospital Planning in an Uncertain World," *Health Care Management Review* 4 (1982): 39–43.

4. Howard L. Smith, Debra A. Thomas, and David J. Ottensmeyer, "Planning Geriatric Services: Considerations and Constraints," *Group Practice Journal,* in press.

# Chapter 5

# Strategic Factors: Management Information Systems

Strategic and tactical planning by hospitals takes place in a vacuum unless accurate data are available for decision making. Given the complexity of prospective reimbursement, it appears that hospitals will be unable to make needed strategic decisions unless they upgrade their information systems. A real dilemma may confront hospital executives who have been reluctant to invest in data management systems. Most management authorities recognize that decisions can be improved through automated information systems, but many hospitals have overinvested in computerized medical records and billing systems, and have underinvested in management information systems. This is a precarious basis for managing prospective payment.

## CAUSES OF UNDERINVESTMENT

Many hospitals have internal automated systems that provide information for operational decisions. Strategic decisions and the information necessary to make those decisions are often omitted from the overall design of these information systems, however. As a result, hospitals have tended to develop very sophisticated information systems for medical record keeping and patient billing. At their greatest extension, these systems may provide basic financial data—balance sheets, expense and revenue statements, pro forma budgets, and the like.

Until the last five years, it was common for hospitals to view themselves as organizations subject to excessive regulation, but also capable of plotting their own destiny. This attitude resulted primarily from retrospective reimbursement, which provided a margin of safety for all hospitals. With minimum attention to cost containment, a hospital could perform without financial risk. If costs increased, charges could be increased. This atmosphere was not conducive to the implementation of a rigorous planning process or of wide-scale control systems designed to increase efficiency.

Hospitals were also reluctant to form alliances with other hospitals, and there were few pressures to encourage multi-institutional arrangements, either to react to new legislation or to manage the rising costs of supplies. Although the tendency to avoid external alliances is clearly breaking down with the pressures created by higher regulation and restricted reimbursement, traditions often prevail.

Hospitals have generally failed to create the type of sophisticated strategic management information systems that would help them address major changes, such as prospective payment, because they have not needed such systems to buttress their strategic management capacities. There has been little pressure to control costs in order to minimize financial risk. There has been little pressure to market services because demand has generally exceeded supply. There has been little pressure to form alliances that counteract regulation. Thus, hospitals have continued to focus their energies on internal operations—not from an analytical/management point of view, but from an operational point of view.

## IMPLICATIONS OF UNDERINVESTMENT

Strategic planning requires an information base on past and current operations. Before long-run decisions can be made, a hospital must know where it has been and where it is going in terms of serving patients. Thus, it is important to be able to determine a hospital's case mix, average length of stay, occupancy, number of patients served, variances in departmental revenues over costs, and similar benchmarks at a given point in time. If these base line patient statistics and financial data were omitted from the hospital's information system, strategic and operational changes could be made only on an intuitive basis. Therefore, even if a hospital has overinvested in operational information systems, at least that investment has provided a basis from which a strategic information system can be developed.

Underinvestment in the operational system places a hospital in a far worse position. With the introduction of prospective payment, such a hospital would discover that it is now confronted with a substantial addition to overhead. Furthermore, there would be no time to fine-tune the system before prospective payment began to have its most substantial impact.

In the best operational computerized information systems, a subsystem channels information to key administrative decision makers—department heads, medical director, chief financial officer, administrator and staff, director of planning, and others. This information aggregates data that might be useful for planning, since administrators are less concerned with a specific patient's episode of care than with the accumulated statistics over a period of time. Yet, many automated systems developed for administrative purposes not only exclude data important for strategic management, but also duplicate data already available on the operating system.

In their haste to adopt new systems, hospitals often overlook the importance of defining which information is needed for which decisions and plans. Unless a hospital has carefully assessed its information needs and analytical programs, it may have two, three, or more vendors supplying hardware, software, and off-site information processing. The essence of a management information system is careful assessment of need, however, not a computerized data set that is equivalent to the state of the art and admired by other hospitals. Unless a management information system contributes to better decisions in the hospital—whether operational or strategic decisions—the investment is of questionable value, and the hospital is merely following fads without a basic plan.

Adoption of computerized technology has always been a problem for hospitals and other large-scale organizations. They have a tendency to invest in the latest technology, expecting that the investment will somehow improve organizational performance. Hospital executives must remember that these automated systems will not replace their own capacity to observe and manage complex situations with a multitude of conflicting and often nonquantifiable variables. Although they may believe that information processing and decision making cannot be improved without the latest in modern technology, the reverse actually occurs more often than not.

The presence of an automated information system may force administrators to adapt their analyses to the system. Many administrators have discovered that the extra piece of information deemed essential for a decision is not retrievable from their system, or, if retrievable, can be obtained only through special programming that involves added expense and time delays. Given the turbulent hospital environment and the premium attached to immediate responses, the ill-conceived, often prepackaged, management information system may quickly become a decision-taking rather than a decision-making system.

This situation is unfortunate under normal circumstances. Hospitals are no longer confronted by normal circumstances, however, but are on the threshold of a revolution in reimbursement. Even if their information-processing needs at the operating and strategic levels had been sophisticated before, they are more complex after the introduction of case mix or prospective reimbursement. Most information systems will not be able to meet the higher demands imposed upon them.

Prospective reimbursement requires an ongoing information system, and it requires such a system immediately. It takes time to modify a functional and effective management information system, much less a substandard data system. Furthermore, it takes at least two years to plan and implement a new decision-oriented management information system. Part of this time must be spent in working out "bugs" that accompany the system. Once the system is fully operational, more time can be devoted to refining operations and integrating programs, routines, and subroutines that were initially omitted.

Hospital executives have some time before the complete phase-in of Medicare prospective reimbursement according to diagnosis-related groups (DRGs). The time and the resources spent in upgrading an inadequate system are detrimental to the strategic management of prospective payment, however. Given the magnitude of the change and the long-run implications of prospective payment, hospitals need to concentrate on managing prospective payment, not on managing their information system.

## MANAGEMENT OF CHANGES

Clearly, the changes wrought by prospective payment will affect both tactical and strategic factors in the hospital. Accurate data on case mix, length of stay, payer revenue, provider productivity, and cost of care have always been valuable in the administration of hospitals. In the past, however, they were only part of the information that administrators might have used to make decisions; now, they will be decision criteria.

The management information system must provide the data needed by hospital staff members who are trying to form strategic and tactical plans for DRG-based reimbursement. Thus, a food service manager who is delegated the responsibility of minimizing cost increases for the forthcoming year must be able to review all food costs, personnel costs, and allocated indirect costs associated with food service. The information must be unambiguous, explicit, and accurate. It should not be necessary for this manager to determine the accuracy of the data or to request additional material on the breakdown of costs or the forecasts of patient demand. Similarly, the director of marketing must be able to target specific markets by analyzing the DRGs that produce more revenues than costs. Not all DRGs will be amenable to marketing strategies—whatever those strategies may be; however, the marketing department may promote some DRGs through education of the medical staff, other DRGs by referral to medical staff members, and still other DRGs by mass media efforts aimed at the general public. Information provided about hospital performance in providing services for these may determine which DRGs are selected for promotion.

Managers at both tactical and strategic levels in hospitals need upgraded information systems in order to plan responses to DRG-based reimbursement. Unless needed information is available early in the management phase, it will be very difficult to formulate either tactical or strategic plans. Furthermore, future plans will be formed around the inadequate plans of the past. In sum, the management information system is the link to critical decision making and planning.

## INFORMATION SYSTEMS VS. DATA SYSTEMS

The various information subsystems that provide data or information for planning, decision making, or control purposes comprise the management information system. Thus, the medical records or billing systems may be one element in the system, but they are not the entire management information system. The focus of a management information system is more than information or data processing; such a system is oriented toward critical, tactical plans and decisions, especially toward strategic management. It is concerned with providing the ingredients that result in good decisions.

There has been considerable debate over the past decade about the broad intentions of management information systems. According to some management authorities, a true information system that can provide data for decisions is but a dream, because information requirements vary significantly.[1] Others imply that the modeling involved in a management information system makes it difficult to capture the intricacies of strategic decision making and, thus, impossible to provide that which managers need most.[2]

If a management information system is to be successful, hospital administrators must clearly define their information requirements. The higher in the hospital hierarchy, the more abstract the information needs. Thus, considerable effort must be devoted to defining specific information needs (i.e., for decisions) and building in flexibility for addressing the inevitable crises that will arise. Information gathering and processing systems alone will not meet the requirements of either department heads or top administrative echelons in hospitals. Information flows that direct meaningful data to them and block meaningless data must be developed.[3] This is difficult work and can seldom be handled completely by an information systems consultant, although hospital executives are often tempted to place themselves in the hands of a consultant.

## INFORMATION NEEDS FOR DRGs

There is nothing really mystical about DRGs. They primarily require hospital executives to analyze performance data according to patient classification. Although there is more emphasis on cost containment, the structure and process of hospital care have not changed. In many respects, the development of DRGs has not introduced anything really new in the way of information requirements; administrators should have been concerned about cost control in the past, and they should be concerned about cost control in the future. Hospital executives must go back to basics in assessing the applicability of their information systems to DRG-based prospective reimbursement, however. They should analyze the strength of their systems in providing decision-oriented data. They should develop a new attitude and a new system design in which data are aggregated around case mix and considered in the key decisions of the hospital.

The data aggregation process should be designed to generate sound indicators of patient utilization for departmental and institutional planning (Figure 5–1). Successive aggregations are produced on an incremental data base until the data are reduced to a series of manageable indicators that administrators can use as key monitoring guidelines. Again, this is hardly a new concept in hospital information management. The implications of this aggregation are new, however; they are a direct result of prospective payment. Administrators, supervisors, and program directors throughout the hospital hierarchy must develop a revised view of operations.

## Incremental Data

Basic incremental data are patient- and diagnosis-oriented. Thus, the file begins with descriptive data on the patient that are key determinants of the DRG rate. This is the obvious purpose in analyzing the information system—to ascertain the building blocks needed for accuracy in reimbursement. Hospitals must ensure that patients are correctly designated; otherwise, reimbursement may be reduced.

Many institutions have failed to utilize fully the patient data at their disposal for institutional planning. In particular, they have begun to plan programs on the assumption that a high percentage of the catchment area population will be interested in a new service. Hospitals have tended to adopt the attitude that any service offered will be used. In many urban areas, this approach has been disastrous for cost containment. Institutionally, more revenues must be generated to support marginal and high-cost programs. Under retrospective reimbursement, this was not a significant problem; under prospective reimbursement, however, this becomes a very significant issue.

Thus, the DRG-oriented information system must serve as a basis for many hospital decisions that, in the past, were based on data generated by the retrospective payment system. The hospital that is contemplating an expansion of its pediatrics program because of a high number of births in its catchment area, for example, might have proceeded on the basis of this awareness alone—that the birth rate has risen. Staff could have been added without much attention to actual population trends, and the hospital could have proceeded to develop the services around new medical staff members. Such an approach now carries a significantly higher risk. The hospital planner must validate the need for the pediatrics program on the basis of patients served, additional patients who may be drawn to the

**Figure 5–1** Aggregating DRG Data

Incremental Data

Patient address data
Demographic data:
  age
  sex
  ethnicity
Admission and discharge dates
DRG number(s)
Attending physician
Referral source
Payers:
  primary
  secondary
Services
Itemized charges
Principal, major and
  secondary diagnoses
Surgical procedures
Surgeon performing the
  principal procedure

Aggregated Data

Case-mix
Average length of stay
Number of patients served
Provider profile
Third-party payer profile

Departmental and Insti-
tutional Planning Centered
Around Patient Mix

program, and, most critically, the financial picture—do the DRGs associated with the program produce more revenues than costs?

Clearly, many other data must be part of an information system centered on patient and case mix data. It is particularly critical to identify the DRG (numbers) services, because a good information system will merge cost data with DRG data to develop profiles of provider expenses per DRG, institutional performance per DRG (for comparison to that of other hospitals), and departmental expenses as a portion of DRG expenses. In addition, it is helpful for hospital executives to know which physicians are primarily responsible for a steady flow of patients through a hospital and what outside sources are referring patients so that the executives can estimate possibilities for expansion of medical staff or of surgical specialties.

Many chief financial officers will acquire subordinate staff members whose primary responsibility is to review financial data on services and itemized charges in order to identify deviances. They must be especially cautious to examine the data for trends:

- Which physicians consistently run over reimbursement for a given **DRG**?
- Is the problem attributable to the entire staff or just one (or two) staff members?
- Have others begun to move toward the mean cost for a given DRG?
- Are there any DRGs that have recently generated higher costs than revenues?

These analytical questions can be answered effectively only if the management information system supporting the analysis is capable of providing timely and accurate information.

Finally, a DRG-oriented information system must incorporate the medical process, which is the essence of DRG reimbursement. The information system must be carefully managed to ensure accuracy of the principal, major, and secondary diagnoses noted. The specific surgical procedures performed, as well as the surgeon performing the procedures, should be specified. In a large hospital with many cases per year, the error potential can accumulate, seriously affecting the level of hospital reimbursement. Thus, the system must have built-in checks that guarantee accuracy.

No one knows how prospective payment systems based on patient mix will evolve over the next decade. It is certain, however, that the use of DRGs will provide third party payers and regulatory agencies with much more data on hospital operations than they have possessed in the past. Because they will be able to develop profiles on each hospital, they will be in a better position to pinpoint DRG creep or other subtle hospital maneuvers to maximize revenue. Therefore, hospitals should adopt a long-run perspective on DRG management. Hospitals will find it easier to establish accurate and legitimate methods from the beginning than to reorient their methods later.

## Aggregated Data

Once the information system has been built around incremental data, routines must aggregate the data into broad indicators. These routines are available with most software packages from the growing number of information processing consultants in the health care field. Many have developed specific packages for DRGs. These packages are certainly more than adequate, if the cautions previously recommended to prevent becoming a captive of the consultant are remembered. If an external consultant is not used, then the hospital probably has a staff capable of programming the routines.

Most hospital administrators, department heads, or program coordinators have neither the time nor the desire to conduct an extensive analysis of performance data—they must rely on the information system to give them convenient surrogates and indexes that convey a large amount of information. The DRG coordinator, the information-processing staff, the financial staff, or the administrative office will handle the specific analysis of performance.

The aggregation of incremental data establishes a working model that focuses a hospital's information system on patient mix. This is only the beginning in constructing the management information system, however. Although the data are specific, they do not address any specific decision issues; they may help hospital executives arrive at a determination, but they do not directly contribute to strategic (and even many tactical) decisions. Another more conceptual level is necessary in the examination of hospital information systems.

## CONCEPTUAL BASIS FOR MANAGEMENT INFORMATION SYSTEMS

In preparation for programming within a management information system, a number of key decisions must be made. A series of questions about the fundamental operating procedures and the strategic concerns of the hospital must be answered. By contemplating answers to these questions and by referring back to the primary decision areas, a hospital should be able to develop a quality flow of information that actually supports rigorous management of DRGs (Figure 5–2).

### Key Decision Areas

The aggregated patient mix data form the hospital's forecast of demand, establishing a point from which the demand for the services of every clinical and

**Figure 5–2** Conceptual Basis for Construction of Management Information System

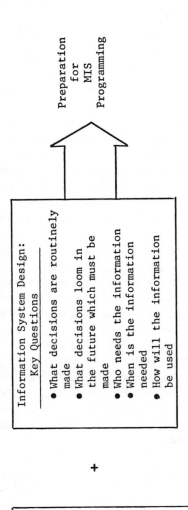

Information System Design:
Key Questions

- What decisions are routinely made
- What decisions loom in the future which must be made
- Who needs the information
- When is the information needed
- How will the information be used

Preparation
for
MIS
Programming

+

Foundation of MIS Design:
Key Decision Areas

- Aggregated Patient Mix Data (Forecast of Demand)
- Financial Plans
  Revenue Budget
  Expense Budget
  Capital Budget
- Marketing Plans
  Retraction of Services
  Expansion of Services
- Planning and Policy
  Management Control
  Program Evaluation
  Organization/Structure
- Human Resource Plans
  Medical
  Nonmedical
- Medical Staff Involvement

ancillary department can be estimated. In the past, hospitals may have been reluctant to use such forecasts as a guide to decision making at the departmental level, because they assumed that the demand would arise or that they could transfer the extra costs to other hospitals (i.e., commercial carriers and private paying patients). Prospective payment destroys this approach to managing. Hospitals will be susceptible to insolvency if they persist in generating more costs than revenues. Therefore, hospitals must forecast patient mix as accurately as possible and plan internal operations around that forecast.

Clinical and ancillary department heads not only must budget according to the forecasted level of patient demand, but also must prepare contingency plans should the budget prove inaccurate. It may be necessary to make plans for retrenchment as well as for expansion. The supervisor, director, or department head's role is certainly much more complex under this new prospective payment mechanism.

Financial plans build on revenue budgets, expense budgets, and capital budgets. Expense budgets acquire additional significance under prospective payment; it is crucial to the success of cost containment that all departments achieve the highest possible level of operating efficiency. Capital budgets are also critical to financial planning under prospective payment. Many authorities have noted the erosion of hospital capital because of the reduction in reimbursement available for these expenses.[4] Increasingly, hospitals have begun to borrow the funds necessary to finance construction or major equipment purchases. This strategy was possible under retrospective reimbursement, because capital costs could be passed on to at least some third parties. The implementation of DRG-based reimbursement may change this manner of thinking, however. Until the management information system has become stable vis-a-vis strategic management information and patient profiles, it may be best to delay plans for construction or major equipment purchases (except for replacement) until staff have analyzed all options. They must be able to define a four-year scenario for funding, given the impending adoption of prospective payment by almost all third parties.

Marketing plans must also be founded on data retrievable from the management information system. Hospitals may decide to expand or retract services on the basis of these data. This is not an unusual approach for many corporations, but hospital corporations have not generally viewed their services in a product line fashion. Except for specialty hospitals, most hospitals perceive themselves as providers of general inpatient care. Now, the management information system must provide objective, financially based data on real or potential patient demand so that executives can decide whether certain services should be deleted.

Staffing is the biggest overhead cost in a hospital. Therefore, costs can almost certainly be reduced or at least maintained in this area. Yet, decisions to encourage higher employee productivity, to reduce turnover, or to expand in a given service area are possible only if the hospital administration has information available on the ramifications of each option. Thus, the management information system must provide the data necessary to forecast the adjusted staffing component in the light of increased or decreased services.

From the planning/policy perspective, the management information system should contribute to extensive management control and program evaluation. It should be compatible with plans to reorganize or at least to assess the organization of services. Although few hospitals are likely to undergo a major reorganization because of prospective reimbursement, many will consider restructuring departments on the basis of cutbacks or group integration to achieve economies of scale.

Last, the management information system must provide information to physicians about their performance. Physicians must make many key decisions under prospective payment, but they will be reluctant to change their behaviors unless they are given explicit information that targets key indexes and suggests alternate action. Physicians, like other hospital staff members, are busy people; thus, the management information system must not overburden them with data. They must be well-informed, however, since they control the medical decisions from which costs are generated.

### Key Questions

Once the key decision areas have been identified, key questions (and subvariations) must be asked in order to structure the required subsystem information. In the marketing decision area, for example, hospital marketing directors routinely decide the following:

- How much should be invested in media (e.g., telecommunications and radio)?
- How much should be invested in personal mailings (e.g., to physicians)?
- What should promotion material contain?
- How long should a promotion campaign last?
- How much should be allowed for planned promotions and how much for emergency promotions (e.g., for a new service that has faltered)?
- How large should the marketing staff be?
- Which services should be highlighted in the forthcoming advertising budget?
- Which marketing efforts should be evaluated?

The hospital marketing area must plan for future decisions as well. This probably involves fewer decisions, but they are also important:

- Can the marketing budget justifiably be enlarged (or reduced) over the next two years, given financial performance in service areas?
- Should marketing attempts be expanded to target more (or fewer) DRGs in the future?

In view of hospitals' uncertain future, the number of decisions that can currently be specified for that future are fairly limited. Hospitals will generally have to observe the trends in prospective payment.

The nature and scope of the information (e.g., detailed facts versus broad trends) required by the marketing department depends largely on whether the director of marketing and development, the chief executive officer, the board of trustees, or marketing staff members will use the information. Similarly, the management information system must be designed to take into account whether the information is needed daily, weekly, monthly, or semiannually.

Finally, the hospital marketing director must ask a series of questions about the way in which the information will be used:

- Will the data be subject to continuing analysis (e.g., in identifying patient origin by ZIP codes for clustering the patient source for various DRGs) in fine-tuning marketing plans?
- Will the data be used for routine evaluations of the marketing effort?
- Will the data be used outside the marketing department (e.g., for strategic planning by the top administrator)?
- Will the data be referred to clinical department heads to underscore various issues in program/department performance vis-a-vis the marketing effort?

## PROBLEMS IN ESTABLISHING A MANAGEMENT INFORMATION SYSTEM

There are significant problems in setting up a management information system to provide data around case mix. Basically, the problems arise because hospitals and software suppliers lack experience in managing DRG-based prospective reimbursement. Fortunately, the existing limitations in creating a prospective payment management information system will decrease as time passes and hospitals (as well as computer system consultants) come to understand the true management information needs of their current environment.

The goal of developing a management information system is to achieve greater internal control of prospective payment perturbations (Figure 5–3). The management information system makes it possible for the administrative staff to concentrate on analyzing case mix–based clinical and cost data and on developing

**Figure 5–3** Missing Ingredients in Prospective Payment Management Information System

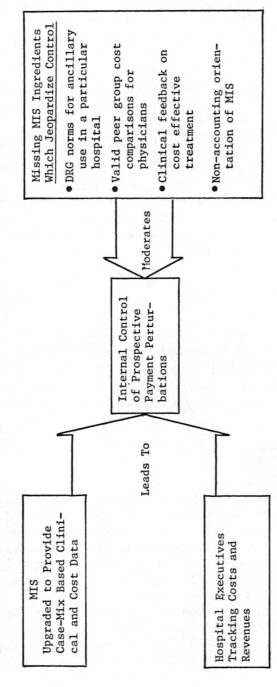

managerial implications from the analysis. Combining these two ingredients—the management information system and management analysis—leads to better performance and, thus, to better internal control over prospective payment effects on the hospital.

The omission of certain ingredients in the formulation of a management information system can moderate and jeopardize that internal control.[5] First, most hospitals will not have enough cases in every DRG to establish a set of norms that are conducive to comparative analysis. (This lack of a statistical base is due in part to the traditional methods of organizing information in an accounting rather than a case mix approach.) For example, it will be difficult to determine whether physicians are overusing ancillary services for some DRGs until the hospital has a sufficient number of cases per year (e.g., more than 10) in each DRG to form a profile. External comparisons may not be valid because they assume that the structure and process of medical care are equivalent from hospital to hospital.

It is also difficult to set a standard for the direct costs that should be assigned to each physician. Valid peer group data for comparison purposes can be derived as more episodes of care are entered into the data profiles, but this does not resolve the problem of the present management of costs. Physicians should not be accused of creating cost containment problems unless it can be proved that costs are actually excessive. The management information system should help resolve this dilemma.

Management information systems in hospitals generally do not provide clinical feedback on cost-effective treatment. This omission is a function of the cost and patient mix orientation of prospective payment. Most information systems in hospitals identify deviances in cost or average length of stay. Although this approach is a useful starting point, it has a negative connotation. A more positive approach would offer alternate courses of action. Thus, physicians not only should be alerted to cases in which they are producing excessive costs, but also should receive some guidance in improving their management of patients through information about prevalent physician practice patterns at the hospital.

Finally, the nonaccounting orientation of a management information system may jeopardize control. Most hospital systems are accounting-oriented, and there is nothing wrong with this orientation if hospitals are to be run simply as business organizations. For many hospitals, this is appropriate. In becoming more efficient—by responding to prospective payment, for example—there is some risk of losing the focus on people as patients, however.

## PHYSICIAN PARTICIPATION IN AN INFORMATION SYSTEM

Because physicians make decisions about care that have substantial ramifications for costs and cost control, it seems unlikely that a hospital can achieve the desired level of control without physician participation in the management information system. Management control practices must be extended to physicians (Figure 5–4).

The management analysis of case mix–based clinical and cost data shows physician performance. That analysis can reinforce the fact that the performance of a physician (or physicians) is exemplary, but the management information system should not stop there. Several strategies for motivating changes in physician behavior can be derived from the development of a DRG-oriented management information system.[6] Four of these ideas involve tactics that are not necessarily data based:

1. education. Once profiles that pinpoint excessively costly DRGs have been developed, continuing education on practice patterns can be provided to the medical staff.
2. administration. Unwanted practice patterns (e.g., ordering an excessive number of laboratory tests) can be reduced by establishing standard operat-

**Figure 5–4** Extensions of Management Practices to Physicians from DRG-Centered Information

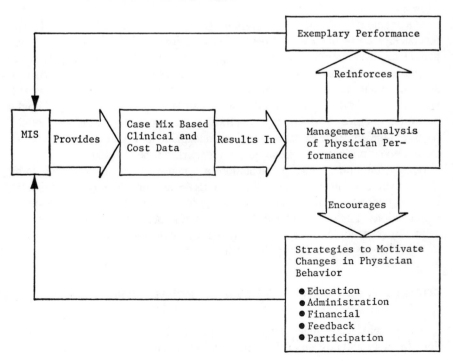

**Table 5–1** Monthly Physician Performance Feedback

| Physician | Historical Cost per Surgical Procedure | Predicted Cost per Surgical Procedure This Month | Differential Change in Efficiency | Total Cost | Total Revenue | Revenue Less Cost |
|---|---|---|---|---|---|---|
| Able | 543.71 | 545.76 | + 2.05 | 2,183.04 | 2,680.00 | + 496.96 |
| Baker | 642.23 | 666.56 | +24.33 | 3,332.80 | 3,350.00 | + 17.20 |
| Coward | 571.64 | 577.20 | + 5.56 | 2,308.80 | 2,680.00 | + 371.20 |
| Druid | 566.72 | 564.19 | − 2.53 | 1,128.38 | 1,340.00 | + 211.62 |
| Ellium | 530.33 | 520.11 | −10.22 | 3,640.77 | 4,020.00 | +1,049.23 |

*Note:* For a similar treatment, see Regina E. Herzlinger and Gordon T. Moore, "Management Control Systems in Health Care," *Medical Care* 11 (1973):416–428.

ing procedures. Physicians might be required to obtain written permission for some tests from their clinical department chairperson.

3. financial risk. Physicians could be placed at financial risk for costs and revenues. If they generate more revenues than costs, they could be allowed to share in the revenues through bonuses. If they generate excessive costs, they could be penalized. It might be possible to terminate a physician from the medical staff for consistent cost abuse.

4. participation. Administrators should use physicians' sense of professionalism to gain their voluntary participation in cost control.

Hospitals should use their management information system as a source of feedback to physicians.[7] Unless physicians know how their costs and their performance compare to those of others, they are unlikely to implement corrective action. Since most physicians are conscientious professionals, they may need no incentive other than this information. They become internally motivated to control their own performance. This requires periodic feedback reports. In Table 5–1, for example, it is apparent that Dr. Baker's costs were excessive this month. Alerted to this deviance by the report, he will probably bring his performance in line with others. He has the greatest motivation possible—his peers are performing at a higher level. In contrast, Dr. Ellium's costs have been consistently below those of the other physicians in her specialty; her historical cost average is the lowest for the group. Specific feedback to this effect may continue to reinforce this behavior. Feedback such as this is the very essence of a functional and supportive management information system.

---

## NOTES

1. John Dearden, "MIS Is a Mirage," *Harvard Business Review* 50(1972):90–99.

2. William Zani, "Blueprint for MIS," *Harvard Business Review* 48(1970):95–100.

3. Richard O. Mason, "Basic Concepts for Designing Management Information Systems" (AIS Research Paper No. 8. Graduate School of Business Administration, UCLA, October, 1969).

4. William O. Cleverly, "Is Hospital Capital Being Eroded under Cost Reimbursement?" *Hospital Administration* 19 (Summer 1974):58–73.

5. Michael Nathanson, "Computers Crank out DRG Cost Data, But How Valid Is Information," *Modern Healthcare* 13 (September 1983):160–164.

6. Ibid.

7. Regina E. Herzlinger and Gordon T. Moore, "Management Control Systems in Health Care," *Medical Care* 9(1973):416–428.

# Chapter 6

# Strategic Factors: Financial Planning

The financial implications of prospective payment are perhaps the most important concern for hospitals. This concern is compounded by the fact that several key financing considerations have yet to be defined. Capital expenses for plant and equipment, for example, have been excluded from the prospective payment system until October 1, 1986.

In many respects, it is appropriate for the underlying structure of prospective payment to be cautiously developed. Hospital planning for current operations and investment in plant and equipment cannot adequately progress while the specifics of the reimbursement regulations are uncertain, however. The possibility of all-payer systems that would require all third party reimbursers to adopt prospective payment confuses planning even further. Given this potential, it is obvious that hospital management staffs must be flexible in developing financial plans through the remainder of the 1980s. On one hand, they must create very specific systems for managing the impact of prospective payment (e.g., adapting medical records and related management information systems). On the other hand, they must avoid establishing strategic plans that overrely on the initial structure of Medicare reimbursement. Although prospective payment systems are likely to multiply among all third parties, hospitals must not overreact.

Considering the magnitude of the effects of prospective reimbursement on hospital financial management, executives must consider several factors in forming a strategic response:

- hospital services/products
- the cost of capital
- capital reimbursement
- capital acquisition
- capital expenditures on equipment

- integration of patients into financing
- prevention of bad debts and the impact of bad debts on financial performance
- charitable care

These critical variables must be well managed if hospitals expect to minimize the adverse impact of prospective reimbursement on the income statement and balance sheet.

Clearly, hospitals must examine the priority of Medicare within their third party reimbursement mix. Hospitals that provide care primarily to patients covered by commercial carriers or Medicaid may opt to retain their standard policies and operating procedures on the ground that it is not worthwhile to revise management methods simply because 5 to 10 percent of their patients rely on Medicare. These hospitals may inadvertently reduce their ability to manage prospective payments successfully, however, should other third parties follow the lead of Medicare. As a result, they could not only overlook the short-run consequences of Medicare, but also could place themselves in a disadvantageous position for managing prospective payments introduced by other third parties. They would not have sufficient experience, nor would their operating systems be capable of handling the new payment environment without extensive upgrading. Hospitals that had already adapted to Medicare would be in a far better position. Although they, too, would be forced to revise procedures, the magnitude of the change would be substantially less.

## HOSPITAL SERVICES/PRODUCTS

Instead of services or patient days, diagnosis-related groups (DRGs) are formed around the resources used in delivering care. Thus, the focus is on the aggregation of services, representing product lines. This eliminates the tendency to group patients whose conditions vary widely in severity and improves hospitals' ability to determine the level of resources invested in any particular patient for a given level of care. The shift to product accounting is one of the major changes associated with DRG-based reimbursement.[1]

The financial implications of this change are very significant because payment is associated with all hospital services rendered for  diagnosis-related care, and the payment is made prospectively. Thus, the major result is the separation of hospital services from physician services. Payment to the hospital is separate from the payment which the physician may receive. The hospital must determine whether it can assemble its resources to provide care while also obtaining an operating surplus.

The strategic ramifications of a shift to product accounting should not be overlooked. Far-reaching changes in hospital control systems may develop. This is not merely an operational switch from one method of accounting to another, but establishes a precedent for accountability in that hospital executives are able to ascertain where and by whom costs and revenues have been generated. The next logical step is to exercise control (i.e., correct deviances). Such an idea is rather revolutionary for clinical and nonclinical staff, who may never have been truly aware of the financial parameters of their performance. The progress of hospital executives toward a more "businesslike" management of their organizations hinges in part on this move to product accounting and accountability for every staff member.

The orchestration of the resource expenditure is responsible for the final financial outcome. If the hospital can control the costs of the aggregation of services, it will have a net profit. Inability to provide a product (i.e., service) that renders a net profit is financially tenuous. If the hospital fails to make a net profit with too many DRGs (i.e., products) or with DRGs for which there are substantial numbers of patients, the outcome may be bankruptcy.

Practically, the shift to a product-based orientation for hospital services has changed financial incentives. Prospective payment has made it necessary to consider costs in any management decision. Furthermore, hospitals will receive essentially the same treatment as far as rate determinations; hence, a hospital's inability to operate within the budgeted rate for each product (i.e., prospective rate for each DRG) will weaken its competitive position. As a consequence, hospital executives must determine whether a product offers a surplus or a deficit by examining the following data:

1. the number and characteristics of patients served
2. the direct resource investment required to deliver the product
3. the indirect investment required to support the delivery of the product
4. the operating margin given reimbursement for the product area[2]

After evaluating the strengths and weaknesses of their product delivery, hospital executives can make plans to improve physician or support personnel productivity, to delete some products, to terminate staff who generate excessive costs, and to make management trade-offs.

## THE COST OF CAPITAL

Financially, the impact of prospective payment on hospitals will be greatest in two areas: current operations and long-run capital investment. The basis for financial solvency is internal control of current operations, but capital investment is also critical to financial success.

The cost of capital must be determined for both indirect and direct services (Figure 6–1).[3] The process by which the cost of capital is determined must be consistent with product accounting and with the DRG-based methods for defining hospital services/products. It is critical that hospitals develop a more refined basis for assigning these capital expenditures to specific treatments, because some hospital products require substantially more sophisticated technology for patient treatment (e.g., radiology for cancer) than do others.

The interest and depreciation on a hospital's investment in plant and equipment must be assigned to the DRGs. Portions of these capital expenses are directly allocated to each DRG. Within the revenue-producing centers, such as the laboratory, radiology department, or pharmacy, capital expense must be incorporated in the charges they assign to patients. Those charges are based on the services/ products delivered. This process is little different from that in cost-based reimbursement, except that costs are no longer simply passed on to the third party. Not

**Figure 6–1** Determining the Cost of Capital under DRGs

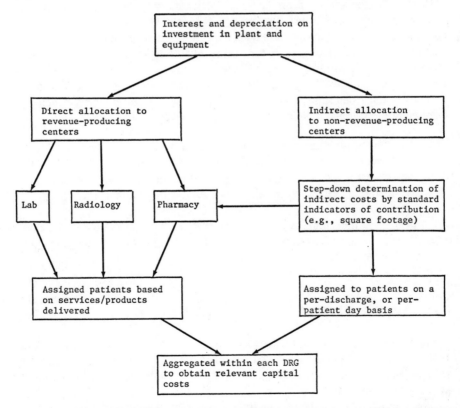

*Source:* Adapted with permission from Michael J. Kalison and Richard Averill, "The Response to PPS: Inside, Outside, Over Time. *Healthcare Financial Management* 1 (1984):82.

only should there be a direct allocation of capital costs under prospective payment, but also there should be a direct allocation of revenue. The final regulations will help clarify these relationships.

The cost of capital can be assigned to non–revenue-producing centers, such as maintenance or administration, by using standardized units in step-down procedures. Again, the costs are ultimately assigned to patients on a per day or per discharge basis. This process of cost allocation is not new; under prospective payment, however, those hospitals in which non–revenue-generating departments require excessive capital investment will be penalized. Thus, hospital executives who want to invest in a costly computer to help in the administration of the facility may discover that the hospital cannot afford such an investment because of the burden placed on revenue-generating departments.

The costs assigned to patients based on services/products delivered and those assigned on a per discharge or per day basis must be aggregated within each DRG so that the hospital can evaluate the cost of capital in relation to the revenue generated. Various management strategies can be initiated at this point in order to keep these costs down, such as

- reducing or deleting services
- delaying investment in new technology
- delaying investment in facility expansion
- terminating plans to expand or to acquire new technology

Clearly, more rigorous thought must be given to all capital investment under prospective reimbursement, because revenue is limited by the prospective payment mechanism.

## CAPITAL REIMBURSEMENT

The reimbursement of health care institutions for capital expenses has generated a great deal of controversy and numerous proposals. Medicare's handling of capital costs will set a new precedent for other prospective payment systems, but Congress delayed until October 1986 the inclusion of capital-related expenses in the Medicare prospective payment rate. For the interim, hospitals are reimbursed for their capital costs on a reasonable cost basis.

Many health care facilities were constructed or modernized between the late 1940s and the 1960s with the assistance of approximately $3.4 billion under the Hill-Burton Act.[4] It has been estimated that $100 to $200 billion will be required to bring hospital facilities up to acceptable operating standards during the next decade.[5,6] This capital will, most likely, come from two main sources: internally generated revenues and external debt. Without a capital reimbursement policy under which each of the major third party payers pays a fair and equitable share of capital expenses, the internally generated revenues will be insufficient to cover both current operations and capital expenses. Debt will then become difficult to obtain, or the cost will be too excessive to consider further expansion. Thus, a fair reimbursement for capital expenses would be the margin that most hospitals require to make a profit.

Payments for capital-related expenses are only a small part of a hospital's total revenues. They amounted to approximately 7.4 percent (including a return on equity) of Medicare reimbursement payments for 1981.[7] Even so, hospitals cannot survive economically over the long run unless they earn a return on invested capital.

Capital-related expenses, based on the reasonable cost method, generally include the following items:[8]

1. net depreciation
2. taxes on land and depreciable assets
3. leases and rentals of depreciable assets
4. betterments and improvements that extend the life at least two years or significantly improve productivity
5. cost of minor equipment capitalized
6. insurance on depreciable assets
7. interest expense on land and depreciable assets
8. return on equity for proprietary providers
9. capital costs of related organizations

## Types of Capital Expenses

Some capital expenses are attributable to major and minor movable equipment; others involve the plant and fixed equipment. Capital expenses for major and minor movable equipment, both clinical and nonclinical, are closely related to operating expenses. The life of this equipment is relatively short; replacement items are generally of the same type and expense, unless they have been technologically improved.

Management must decide the amount and type of equipment to be replaced by labor (and vice versa). It is relatively easy to change the emphasis in the uses of hospital equipment because of its short depreciable life. There are strong incentives to substitute capital for labor under the current Medicare capital reimbursement policy, since labor expenses are treated as operating costs and are subject to reimbursement limits. This is also true in the initial phases of DRG-based prospective reimbursement. Furthermore, it probably characterizes most other third party payers that use prospective reimbursement for operating costs and cost-based reimbursement for capital expenses.

Capital expenses associated with the plant, fixed equipment, and land involve long-term investments. The physical plant cannot be converted to other uses without substantial capital expenditures and, normally, numerous reviews from many public regulatory agencies prior to approval. The basic community need for the facility should be demonstrated prior to construction. This type of capital expense often requires Section 1122 approval or a certificate of need in order to qualify for Medicare reimbursement.

## Proposals for Capital Reimbursement

Medicare appears to be the leader in prospective payment. Hospitals will probably gear their charge systems to Medicare's reimbursement policy, because it provides a significant portion of their revenues. Medicaid, which is likely to follow Medicare's reimbursement policy, is the second highest source of revenue for many hospitals; Medicare and Medicaid, together, account for approximately 40 percent of all hospital revenues.

A number of health care organizations have *proposed* various methods for including capital-related expenses in Medicare's prospective payment system. The major points of these proposals are outlined below. Since the content of any of these proposals may vary at any given point in time, please contact the relevant organization for a precise definition of its current position on Medicare's capital reimbursement. The proposals have been summarized below in the interest of showing the trends in proposed capital reimbursement strategies advocated by leading health care organizations. Again, hospital executives are interested both in the specific elements of each proposal and (most importantly) in the implications of these proposals for other third party payers who may also adopt prospective payment. When this occurs, the debate surrounding capital reimbursement will surface once again.

1. Healthcare Financial Management Association (HFMA)[9]

   - Equipment-related costs—major movable and minor equipment—would be included in the prospective reimbursement payment. The total prospective payment would be updated annually by the hospital market basket index and adjusted for technological advances. This would permit hospital executives to use their judgment in capital-labor trade-offs.
   - Plant-related costs would be reimbursable on a fair share basis to include a return on equity for for-profit hospitals. Future plant investment would require Section 1122 approval or a certificate of need. This portion of capital expense would be added to the prospective payment and updated annually as a separate part of the payment.

- No transition period would be required, as the basis for reimbursement of the plant-related portion of capital expense would be the same as it is now.

2. American Hospital Association (AHA)[10]

- All capital costs would be incorporated into the Medicare prospective payment, providing the same incentives for cost-effective decisions on capital-related expenses as are provided for decisions on operations-related expenses.
- Capital-labor mix and debt-equity decisions would be based solely on their cost-effectiveness, rather than partly on the reimbursement method.
- The control and financial predictability of capital costs would be improved both for hospitals and the payer.
- A return for capital would be included in the prospective payment, using an industrywide cost average during the initial year. Both capital and operating expenses would be updated annually, using the hospital market basket index.
- A separate factor for technology would be applied annually.
- There would be a transition period in which hospitals would elect either to have all costs included in the Medicare reimbursement rate or to continue under the current cost-based system for a specific period. The hospital would make this choice based on current plans for major capital expenditures In the transition period, for example, the hospital would elect to remain under the cost-based system until any ongoing construction was completed in order to obtain a higher reimbursement rate.

3. National Committee for Quality Health Care (NCQHC)[11]

- Capital-related costs would be budget-neutral. Capital payments would be based on historical costs and would require no transition period.
- Capital costs would be incorporated into DRG costs at a flat percentage of the DRG rate. This figure would be inflated annually by the market basket index, which includes a capital component.
- Capital-related costs would be adjusted according to the hospital-specific weighted average age of the capital assets. The weighting method would minimize the redistribution of capital funds among hospitals as a result of their particular point in the capital cycle.

Although Anderson and Ginsburg do not recommend a specific method for capital reimbursement under the prospective payment system, they do address three basic problems associated with a capital reimbursement policy:[12]

1. It is difficult to determine the amount of reimbursement in the aggregate. The issue involved is not only whether the payment system is fair, but also whether a hospital's investment is the correct amount to provide adequate medical care for a community.

2. Once the aggregate amount of reimbursement has been determined, the best way to distribute capital reimbursement to hospitals must be found. Two types of reimbursement have been proposed. One is an industrywide rate that would be added to the prospective payment rate for operating costs. The other is a specific rate tailored to each hospital's unique circumstances.

3. Transition problems are likely to arise, no matter which approach is taken. An industrywide approach favors older hospitals, since an industry average rate would lag behind the actual rate and hospitals that are new or that are expanding or renovating would be burdened with a debt that would probably be higher than the industry average. The hospital-specific approach favors newer hospitals, which would recoup more reimbursement for capital costs during the beginning years of the repayment period than the actual cost of the repayment and interest. The reimbursement for capital costs for older facilities would be much lower, probably less than the actual cost of the mortgage payments. This could preclude older facilities from building a reserve for future construction or improvements.

Noting these difficulties, Anderson and Ginsburg suggested that a split method would solve many of the problems—prospective reimbursement for equipment and the cost-based reimbursement for the plant and fixed assets.

## Overview of Capital Reimbursement

The methods of reimbursing hospitals for capital-related expenses under DRG-based reimbursement are founded on the assumption that the Medicare DRG-weighting factor is indicative of the actual costs incurred by a hospital in performing that service. It is also generally assumed that equipment and facilities will be used in the same consistent proportion.

Some of the proponents of a single reimbursement payment that takes into account both operating costs and capital-related expenses contend that market forces will determine the right price for hospital services. Unfortunately, the health care industry's pricing policies have little to do with market forces. The patient generally does not select the hospital; the physician does. Patients who have insurance coverage generally do not care what hospital they use; normally, they pay only a small portion of the total bill. Those who cannot afford to pay usually receive care from public assistance, charity, or county hospitals.

The portion of capital expenses attributable to movable major and minor equipment should be included in each prospective reimbursement rate, because much of the capital equipment is related to the provision of services to patients. The equipment is replaced periodically with new and improved equipment, depending on management decisions, available funds, technological advances, and the labor market climate. The equipment purchased may or may not be labor-intensive. Switching from labor-intensive practices to capital-intensive equipment should not be determined by reimbursement procedures, but by clinical, cost, and efficiency factors. If equipment costs are factored into the reimbursement rate, however, an acceptable utilization rate for the equipment should be established. In any system in which cost containment is an objective, as it is in the prospective payment system, it seems only logical that utilization should be considered.

The second part of the capital equation, capital expenses for plant, fixed equipment, land, and all costs related to them, should be reimbursable through a cost-based system.

In considering facility expansion, new facility construction, or renovation of existing facilities, health care planners must take into account the current and future utilization rate (percent of occupancy). An increasing utilization rate might be considered a requirement for approval, especially in growing communities, rural areas, and in some intercity areas. This permits hospitals to construct, finance, and receive payment for facilities that approach optimum economic efficiency. This portion of capital expenses should be shared among all third party payers of inpatient services.

Utilization of the facility, however, must be taken into consideration when the facility is built or renovated. At that time, estimates of the utilization must be considered and approved by the proper agencies via Section 1122, CON, or some other authority. This assumes, of course, that a state has an effective regulatory agency which could undertake this sort of analysis. The depreciation and other related capital expense should be pro rated to all patients based on the expected utilization or a range for the utilization with a set maximum and minimum. Hospitals could add a surcharge for facility capital expense to their bills for outpatient care.

Hospitals that maintain a utilization rate between a set minimum and a set maximum would not be rewarded or penalized. Those that maintain a rate above the maximum would be rewarded; those that fall below the minimum would be penalized. In addition, as more debt financing is used for the construction and renovation of facilities, hospitals' knowledge that reimbursement is assured for the physical structure—provided that they exceed the minimum utilization rate—should make the acquisition and cost of debt financing more accessible.

The capital expense for plant and fixed equipment could be computed as a daily charge per room:

$$\frac{\text{Capital Expense}}{\text{Total Number Rooms} \times \text{Utilization} \times 365} = \text{Room Charge}$$

On the other hand, the capital expense could be included in the prospective payment rate, based on a percentage of the reimbursement rate, provided that the length of stay or some other factor(s) can be correlated with the DRG weighting. The AHA has examined the relationship between current Medicare DRG weights for operating costs and other factors that might correlate with capital expenses. A high correlation was found between DRG weights and the use of facilities and equipment; the higher the DRG weight, the more capital resources used.[13]

The daily capital expense charge could also be calculated from the average DRG-weighting index (ADWI) of the hospital for the previous year. The average cost per admission per DRG weight of 1.000 would be

$$\frac{\text{Total Inpatient Billed Charges}}{\text{ADWI} \times \text{Total Admissions}} = \frac{\text{Billed Charge}}{\text{Admission}}$$

The percentage factor would be

$$\frac{\text{Total Capital Expense (Pro Rated to Inpatient)}}{\text{Total Inpatient Billed Charge}} = \% \text{ Increase}$$

This percentage would then be added to the DRG prospective rate. Of course, the total inpatient billed charges would have to be those from the previous year. Alternately, a six- or 12-month moving average could be used.

Capital expenses could be, for the most part, precalculated. Either method would probably suffice, as capital expenses are only a small part of a hospital's total expenses. The overall percentage of error in calculating the actual capital cost per DRG, as a percentage of total cost, on a per capita basis, or by length of stay would have little effect on total hospital costs.

Generally, the hospitals most affected by capital financing policies are facilities with a high ratio of capital costs to operating expenses. These hospitals tend to be for-profit, since nonprofit and government-owned hospitals have relied less on debt financing in the past.[14,15] Hospitals that have added beds since the late 1970s, when interest rates were very high, may also have a high ratio of capital costs to operating expenses. It appears that the thrust of the problem then, is how to be equitable and fair to all parties involved under Medicare and future prospective payment systems. It must be ensured that sufficient facilities are available, health care costs remain reasonable, quality care is provided, and that the capital base of the hospital system remains viable for the future.

Hospitals and other health care facilities should not be permitted to shift any underpayments that result from one third party payer's policy to the other payers. Therefore, any system that is implemented must be uniform for all. The system must distinguish movable major and minor equipment capital expenses. Fixed plant capital expenses, fixed equipment, facilities, land, and all expenses related to them are approved, in most cases, by public agencies in order to ensure that the needs of the community are met. Within certain limits, the estimates of both the institution and the approving regulatory agency must be based upon available demographic information relating to the needs of the community for health care facilities. It appears that these suggestions would provide fair reimbursement for capital costs while minimizing the financial incentives to initiate unneeded new construction or elaborate purchase arrangements (or similar strategies) that might raise the cost of capital. Management would have control over the daily operations of the hospital and would base all operational financial decisions on cost-effectiveness, not on reimbursement policies. The facility cost would be reimbursable, thus ensuring that hospitals are available to meet the community's needs now and in the future.

Given the recent changes in capital availability, the erosion of capital in the hospital industry, and the growth of for-profit chains, the decision on capital financing is of obvious importance. For most hospitals, it is best to build strategic plans on these financial constraints and to plot strategy according to the announcements by third party payers about their intended adoption of prospective reimbursement.

Others suggest that hospitals must forge their destiny, regardless of the reimbursement climate, because hospital services will always be needed. If third party payment for capital expenditures is insufficient to cover the costs associated with inevitable replacement or renovation, hospitals could eventually go bankrupt anyway. Therefore, say the advocates of this approach, it is best to proceed without focusing excessively on current events in reimbursement or without planning the construction of facilities to capitalize on some advantageous niche or loophole in ensuing reimbursement structures. Such a view may simply be an excuse for not asking and answering the most difficult questions in the hospital field, however.

Finally, hospital executives should remember that the most important issue is the ability of their institutions to generate profits under prospective reimbursement. They should not overconcentrate on capital costs, which represent a single digit percentage of all costs, only to lose control of operating costs. A balanced perspective is appropriate and necessary. DRG payments and inflation factors that raise those payments remain the strategic financial variables for most hospitals.

## CAPITAL ACQUISITION

The prospective payment limitations on capital reimbursement may increase the financial risk for hospital investors. Hospitals now will have to show investors that they can run operations efficiently and can meet the long-term debt obligations that they have acquired. Given their past failure to control costs, some hospitals may have a very difficult time convincing lending institutions that they have amended their practices and are therefore able to service debt. This situation is compounded further by the possibility that regulatory agencies will restrict the DRG rate, the inflation factor built into that rate, or the manner (i.e., formula) in which they reimburse hospitals for capital expenses. Since hospitals have no control over the rates and lending institutions will quickly be apprised of the situation, it may become exceptionally difficult for hospitals to obtain the capital support that they need. Their ability to carry a debt will diminish with the prospective payments.

Hospitals are increasingly being rejected in their search for new capital.[16] Approximately 50 percent of all hospitals are estimated to be marginal in their capacity to service debt. With only 16 to 20 percent of all hospitals rated by Standard and Poor, it is very clear that hospitals are no longer considered the investment that they once were. One conclusion is inevitable—hospitals have a very difficult financial future in front of them. If hospitals cannot borrow equity, they cannot upgrade facilities that have deteriorated. If the facilities deteriorate sufficiently, hospitals will be unable to attract patients, particularly insured patients who do not create bad debts. It is difficult for hospitals whose resources are already stretched too thin to circumvent these events.

There is an exception to this scenario, at least for the short run. Hospitals that belong to chains or join consortiums have retained earnings or other resources for loans. For-profit hospital chains are most likely to survive under these conditions, but they are not guaranteed access to capital. The key to capital acquisition has always been good credit—the ability to pay debts. This ability will receive closer scrutiny under prospective payment.

Kalison, Averill, and Webb suggested that the new prospective payment environment will offer substantial access to capital if the correct outside response is implemented.[17] In their model, hospitals must carefully manage

1. volume (i.e., number of patients)
2. case mix (i.e., allocation of patients to DRGs)
3. cost control
4. revenue

By assessing the strengths and weaknesses of their hospital along these four parameters, hospital executives can introduce revenue flows that allow the servicing of debt. The low risk associated with the loan will help hospitals find new sources of capital. In some cases, the source of capital will not be a loan, but a new multi-institutional relationship.

## CAPITAL EXPENDITURES ON EQUIPMENT

In view of the greater constraints on revenue, prospective payment may alter traditional methods of purchasing and leasing equipment. Wasserman described the results of the New Jersey experiment in prospective payment and equipment investment:

- The criterion of clinical applicability was usually supplemented by other criteria.
- Economic considerations (e.g., productivity and efficiency), in addition to clinical applicability, were often the dominant concerns.
- Equipment was evaluated for its marketing potential.
- Requests for new equipment, including physician-initiated requests, were carefully screened.
- Equipment was assessed for its additional requirements in investment (e.g., personnel).[18]

This rethinking about the adoption of medical technology may lead to significant changes in the diffusion of technological innovation.

The problem in applying the New Jersey results to other prospective payment systems is, of course, the extent to which the New Jersey system is replicated in other states. Because the New Jersey model was adopted in conjunction with operational changes in the current Medicare policy, however, it provides fairly accurate data on anticipated changes in hospitals that are interested in modifying their internal operations because of a high percentage of Medicaid patients in the payer mix.

Most dramatic is the incorporation of evaluation criteria (for equipment purchase or lease) that are nonmedical in nature. Hospitals will become increasingly responsible for addressing the significant economic issues—efficiency, productivity, and external investment—in equipment purchases. Physicians will become increasingly responsible for validating the economic return from their proposed investments. This is a minor revolution for hospitals and medical staff members who have previously been able to evaluate investments in equipment on the sole basis of medical efficacy. The inclusion of other criteria, however, presents a unique opportunity for the clinical staff to become more sensitive to the cost control issues with which they must live in the future.

The interest in the marketing potential of equipment in New Jersey hospitals was a new development. In the past, the marketing potential of equipment has been rather limited. Recently, however, with substantial investment in new radiological technology (e.g., computerized axial tomography [CAT] scanners and nuclear magnetic imagers), equipment has really become an important ingredient of marketing programs. Thus, technology not only defines a hospital's line of services or products, but also becomes a focal point around which marketing messages are centered.

Equipment is now being assessed in terms of the supporting resources required to run, maintain, and obtain the maximum benefit from it. Although these supporting costs are usually variable rather than fixed, the difference between fixed and variable costs diminishes as long as the equipment is being used. A more important concept is productivity. Equipment and the personnel who use it must be highly productive in order to drive down costs. This effect of productivity will increase the debate over capital investment versus labor investment. In this case, the forces may favor the human element, since the fixed investment in people is less. Therefore, hospitals may have greater flexibility by not making a long-run capital investment in equipment.

## INTEGRATION OF PATIENTS INTO FINANCING

With the implementation of DRGs and prospective payment, it may be necessary for patients to become involved in the financing of medical care. Patients have been fairly well protected from the financial responsibility for their medical care with the growth of third party reimbursement. Yet, health insurance premiums have placed significant burdens on both individuals and their employers. Business coalitions represent one prevailing reaction to high health care costs. Business coalitions are promoting wellness programs for employees—changing health insurance benefits, expanding co-insurance and deductibles, and undertaking self-insurance. In some cases, health care consumers are being asked for help in the problem of containing costs.

An original way to integrate patients into the financing of care—other than the traditional co-insurance and deductibles—is to reimburse them for remaining well. Some employers have observed that employees have no financial incentive to avoid illness. Thus, an increasing number of businesses are self-insuring employees, offering financial incentives for employees who minimize health care expenditures in a given year.

Hospitals must also become more innovative in order to integrate patients into the financing of care. Cost shifting will be increased unless systems that apply to all payers are implemented in all states. Since it will undoubtedly be some years before a universal system is fully implemented (if ever), hospitals will probably encounter significant backlash from patients who discover discrepancies between charges to their insurance carrier and those to other third party payers or themselves. Such problems can be minimized by establishing separate reporting/billing forms for different payer classifications. This, of course, will necessitate a higher investment, and some hospitals may not want to make such an investment. It should be balanced, however, against the added investment required for billing clerks and other personnel to explain discrepancies in billing.

## BAD DEBTS AND FINANCIAL PERFORMANCE

Often than shifts in reporting or shifts in deductibles/co-insurance by third parties to integrate patients into medical care financing, prospective payment should have a minimal impact on the bad debt structure of a hospital. Because of the increased emphasis on cost containment, however, it is very likely that hospitals will place greater emphasis on accounts receivable. The leniencies of the past should disappear.

It is difficult for most hospitals to manage bad debts. Unfortunately, prospective payment does not provide a hospital with any additional leverage to obtain payment. They must continue to pursue traditional avenues for collecting bad debts, such as the use of credit and collection agencies. Bad debts place hospitals in a disadvantageous position in regard to controlling costs, however. Refusing to provide care to marginal credit cases could minimize bad debts and hold down costs, but hospitals' reputations may suffer in the process.

## CHARITABLE CARE

Depending on the payer mix, prospective payment may present extreme difficulties to hospitals that provide a significant amount of charitable care. This is most likely to be the plight of public hospitals, since one easy way for a hospital to contain costs will be to provide care only to those who will pay all or at least a significant portion of their bills and to refer charitable care patients to other hospitals—undoubtedly public hospitals.

Legislation on DRGs and public hospitals continues to evolve. It appears that public hospitals (e.g., county hospitals) may have to be subsidized from local sources. Congress has not yet enacted any special legislation that would compensate public hospitals for their heavy load of charitable cases. This is a dangerous predicament, because the problem will grow worse rather than better. These hospitals with a heavy load of charity patients clearly *must* heighten productivity and control costs.

## NOTES

1. Marilyn Mannisto: "Managing Case-Mix Reimbursement," *Trustee* 36 (1983):30–32.

2. Steven F. Kukla and Henry J. Bachofer, "Prospective Pricing: Advice and Warnings," *Trustee* 37 (June 1983):38.

3. Michael J. Kalison and Richard Averill, "The Response to PPS: Inside, Outside, Overtime," *Healthcare Financial Management* 1 (January 1984):78–88.

4. Richard W. Furst, *Financial Management for Health Care Organizations* (Boston: Allyn & Bacon, 1981).

5. Gerald Anderson and Paul B. Ginsburg, "Prospective Capital Payments to Hospitals," *Health Affairs* 2 (Fall 1983):52–63.

6. Charles Bradford, George Caldwell, and Jeff Goldsmith, "The Hospital Capital Crisis: Issues for Trustees," *Harvard Business Review* 60 (1982):56–67.

7. Healthcare Financial Management Association, "Proposed Method of Medicare Payment for Hospital Capital-related Costs" (Revised exposure draft, January, 1984).

8. *Federal Register,* vol. 48, 39,752, September 1, 1983.

9. Healthcare Financial Management Association, "Proposed Method of Medicare Payment."

10. American Hospital Association, "Incorporating Capital Costs into Medicare Prospective Payment Prices" (Draft, July, 1983).

11. National Committee for Quality Health Care, "Proposed Methods for Incorporating Capital-related Costs within the Medicare Prospective Payment System" (Draft, January, 1984).

12. Anderson and Ginsburg, "Prospective Capital Payment to Hospitals."

13. American Hospital Association, "Payment for Capital under Medicare: An Analysis of Options" (Chicago: December, 1983).

14. Mark Tatge, "Industry Execs Unhappy with Capital Proposals," *Modern Healthcare* 14 (1984): 28–29.

15. Cynthia Wallace, 'New Proposals Complicate Debate," *Modern Healthcare* 14 (1984):28–30.

16. "Two-thirds of U.S. Hospitals Facing Capital Market Limits," *Hospitals* 57 (1983):57.

17. Michael J. Kalison, Richard F. Averill, and Richard J. Webb, "The Outside Response," *Healthcare Financial Management* 14 (1984):92–99.

18. Jeffrey Wasserman, "Lessons from New Jersey," *Hospitals* 57 (1983):66–68.

# Chapter 7

# Strategic Factors: Cost Containment and Management Control

The goal of prospective payment is to establish an incentive for efficient operations.[1] Since prospective payment places hospitals at a financial risk if they exceed the planned reimbursement rate, greater efforts must be made internally to contain costs and thereby maintain financial solvency. The problem is primarily managerial in nature—management must control the efforts of medical and nonmedical providers in order to achieve efficiency.

## INCENTIVES UNDER PROSPECTIVE PAYMENT

Most proponents of prospective payment systems assume that these systems create sufficient financial incentives to motivate operating efficiency. By incorporating cost consciousness into the current and future budgeting, planning, and decision-making processes, hospitals should be able to keep costs below reimbursement rates. If the hospital fails to achieve efficiency, it will suffer a financial loss; if it achieves efficiency, it will have a balanced budget or a surplus.

The simple fact that a hospital is at financial risk under prospective payment does not mean that its operations will become efficient, however.[2] Hospitals may continue inefficient delivery patterns under prospective payment. This system may result in elaborate accounting and budgeting maneuvers to confound the reimbursement system, as well as adjustments in the case mix, number of cases, and length of treatment patterns.[3] These unintended consequences are especially prevalent in hospitals that have a diversity of reimbursement sources and variance in case mix severity. With Medicare's implementation of prospective reimbursement based on diagnosis-related groups (DRGs), a hospital that has a substantial patient load covered by Blue Cross and private insurance is in a better position if it does *not* operate at optimum efficiency. Since these third party payers may not fall under the prospective rate umbrella, deficits accrued under the prospective rate can be recovered from them. Furthermore, a dual system of patient care may evolve in which care provided under prospective reimbursement is less intense than that provided under other reimbursement methods.

The success of prospective reimbursement programs in controlling hospital expenditures is mixed. The early evaluations that helped generate research methods were moderated by significant environmental changes (e.g., an economic stabilization program) that ultimately influenced the results.[4] Later evaluations have indicated that prospective payment is effective in minimizing hospital costs, as seen in lower expenditures per patient day, per admission, and per capita.[5] The way in which these reimbursement programs have actually achieved cost control remains unclear, however.

Hospitals have for the most part overlooked the role of internal management practices in hospital efficiency and quality of care.[6] For example, studies of prospective reimbursement in hospitals typically focus on economic outcomes. Less emphasis has been given to *how* lower costs are attained. As a consequence, the health care field has yet to form a viable theory of management control as it relates to health care costs.[7]

## MANAGEMENT CONTROL AND DRGs

The impact of DRGs must be managed (i.e., controlled) by hospital executives, who are ultimately responsible for translating DRGs into operational plans and for ascertaining that fiscal performance is maintained. The board of trustees is concerned with critical management decisions and the implementation of those decisions, but the board's overall orientation is above the operating level. The medical staff is more interested in the provision of medical services and quality of care than in the success of cost containment efforts in providing those services. Thus, management control remains in the hands of hospital executives.

Management control can be defined as the regulation of services in accordance with the requirements of plans. The steps involved in the control process include

- establishing standards
- measuring performance
- comparing actual results with standards
- correcting deviations from standards[8]

Health care facilities that monitor performance and correct deviations will eventually observe improvements in the efficiency with which services are provided. This is especially true for facilities that are functioning under prospective payment, since the budgeting incentive provided by the prospective rate reinforces the management control processes.

In view of this definition of control, it can be said that there are two main dimensions of control in containing hospital costs under DRGs:

1. standard setting and monitoring of standards
2. implementation of policies to improve outputs for a given investment of resources

These ideas are related to key hospital staff members in Table 7–1.

**Board of Trustees**

The support of the board of trustees for cost containment efforts must be highly visible throughout the hospital. The board's commitment to cost control policies must be unwavering; otherwise, there will be little interest shown by key hospital personnel. Without this commitment of the hospital's highest authority, hospital executives will discover that their action plans are neglected or ignored. It will be difficult to motivate employees, and the structure of tactical plans will give way to half-hearted efforts and substandard performance.

The board of trustees must take an active role in setting standards—that is, expectations—and acknowledging performance that meets or exceeds those cost containment benchmarks. In this sense, the board can become involved not only in setting standards, but also in monitoring performance. Certainly, the board should

---

**Table 7–1** Contribution of Hospital Staff Members to DRG Cost Control

| | Contribution to Main Dimensions of DRG Cost Control | |
|---|---|---|
| *Source of Control* | *Standard Setting and Monitoring of Standards* | *Implementation of Policies To Improve Outputs* |
| Board of trustees | High | Low |
| Hospital administration | High | High |
| Medical staff | Medium | High |
| Ancillary staff | Low | High |

*Note:* The extent to which each source contributes to the cost control dimensions has been inferred from the work of R. Herzlinger ("Can We Control Health Care Costs?" *HBR* 56, March-April 1978, p. 109); J.E. Harris ("Regulation and Internal Control in Hospitals" *Bulletin of N.Y. Academy of Medicine* 55, 1979, p. 8); and R.E. Allison ("Administrative Responses to Prospective Reimbursement," *Topics in Health Care Financing* 3, Winter 1976, p. 97).

not become excessively mired in the detail of control, but it must show the hospital staff that it has a working knowledge of where performance is, and is not, meeting expected performance levels. The board must convey this awareness through the hospital administrator, even though the urgency of cost control may justify greater involvement of the board at the operational level.

There are many strategies for achieving board visibility, and each hospital must choose a strategy consistent with the uniqueness of its particular situation—past cost control efforts, personalities of staff, and past commitment of the board to major strategies and tactics. For example, a board of trustees may support cost control efforts through special memos to all department heads or through special staff meetings in which at least one board member is present to discuss the interests of the board. The board may also construct a system of quarterly bonuses to acknowledge the efforts of individuals or departments that have performed in an exemplary fashion.

The board of trustees makes a lesser contribution to the implementation of policies that improve cost control outputs within the hospital. Because the board remains interested in the broad picture, it should concentrate on advising the management staff about the formulation of goals and tactics without becoming overly involved in their implementation.

## Hospital Administration

Hospital administrators work closely with the board of trustees in setting standards for cost control and monitoring performance according to those standards. Most hospital administrators realize that they serve as the operating agent for the board of directors, but few really combine the strategic management and operational interests of their positions. Even though standards are set, they may not be effectively controlled (i.e., monitored) because the press of daily decisions limits the time available to administrators to manage systematically.

The importance of hospital administrators' contribution to the implementation of policies that improve outputs has long been understood, but the notion of control—monitoring performance and correcting deviances—has been neglected, except in the most critical areas of funding and quality. Effective management control for cost containment begins and ends with a well-structured, flexible, and pervasive control system that identifies and corrects poor performance. The integrity of the control system depends on a commitment to performance review and meaningful action that corrects deficiencies in operations.

## Medical Staff

Although the medical staff works with the hospital administrator and board of trustees in setting standards and monitoring performance for cost containment, the medical staff's involvement in the management control process is usually superficial. The need for medical staff participation in the implementation of policies to improve outputs highlights this deficiency. Several reasons can be identified for this discrepancy. Some authorities have suggested that management cost control systems have failed to place physicians at risk for excessive costs in the production of hospital services.[9,10] Other authorities point to physicians' lack of knowledge about the need to control costs.[11,12] Whatever the reason, the medical staff must participate in cost control policy implementation because medical decisions determine which hospital services are provided to patients.

**Ancillary Staff**

It is clear that ancillary staff members, such as those in the housekeeping, laundry, food service, billing, and maintenance departments, can make little contribution to the setting of cost control standards and monitoring of those standards. Some ancillary personnel, such as nurses, laboratory technicians, radiology technicians, and therapists, may be more involved, however.

There is growing evidence that the best control is that implemented at the point of production. If this principle is applicable to medical care, it is possible that the ancillary staff should be involved in standard setting to a greater extent than that normally found in past hospital operations. Monitoring of performance levels is unlikely to deviate from past patterns, however. Unfortunately, because there has been no system of rewards that links productivity and cost control to performance by ancillary staff in hospitals, managers have had less motivation to establish meaningful cost control standards or to monitor performance.

Obviously, the ancillary staff members must be concerned about the implementation of cost control policies that improve their output. Although many staff members may incorporate this concern into their professional identification, hospital executives should not rely on self-direction for the attainment of cost containment. A plan to control must be formed at the top echelons of the hospital. This plan must encompass all operating levels, yet permit flexibility for the more spontaneous cost containment efforts that are developed at those levels.

## INDUCING MANAGEMENT CONTROL

Herzlinger,[13] and Herzlinger and Moore[14] have argued for improved management control systems in health care organizations. Their ideas reflect the theory that cost control relies on the provision of better information to administrative and clinical decision makers. They suggested that hospitals must

1. increase the application of business methods to nonclinical departments
2. develop information systems that provide data for decision making to both administrative and clinical staff
3. utilize multi-institutional arrangements, such as group purchasing plans

Cleverly and Mullen noted that suggestions such as these are conceptually sound, but offer little practical guidance to hospitals.[15] Problems in creating specific cost containment practices have already been observed in nursing homes.[16] A more universally applicable model of inducing cost control is needed.

**Incentives**

From a management control perspective, it appears that the best method for achieving cost control is to provide incentives that motivate desired behavior.[17] Costs can be reduced only when staff—both clinical and nonclinical—have some reason for pursuing cost control. Such systems must build directly on human behavior and human expectations. Today, the pressure generated by excessive health care expenditures has permitted a more liberal attitude toward cost control.

Cleverly and Mullen have recently suggested an entrepreneurial approach to cost containment that incorporates the use of economic incentives.[18] Appropriately motivating incentives for top hospital executives could include

- stock options
- stock ownership
- compensation linked to profit
- bonus systems

Clearly, the first three are most applicable to private, for-profit ventures. Yet, even nonprofit facilities can participate in bonus systems if the definition of bonus is creative. This is the key—the board of directors must be creative in designing compensation plans. Such creativity can then filter down through the administrative ranks.

Smith, Ottensmeyer, and Pasternak noted that incentive compensation plans, such as that recommended by Cleverly and Mullen, can also be applied to a hospital's medical staff, although they questioned whether voluntary regulation of health care costs through incentive compensation systems is most appropriate for hospital cost containment.[19] Medical groups have a wide variety of physician payment plans, but the problem of compensating physicians who are not employees of hospitals, merely staff members, remains. Hospitals are already experiencing a cost dilemma, and adding physicians into the variable cost overhead may complicate matters. The more appropriate criterion, however, is the amount saved through the incentive compensation plan. So, there may be room for incentive compensation in the long run.

Smith, Ottensmeyer, and Pasternak also pointed out that physicians, like other professionals, are motivated by a complex ensemble of factors, only some of which are economically oriented. Physicians are often so economically self-sufficient that they need not trade off quality and cost of care. They may forego economic gain to provide a pattern of treatment (and possibly an amenity level) that approaches the highest quality of care. These behaviors and attitudes may have been engrained from years of practice under more liberal payment and reimbursement systems. The marginal benefit in dollars that these physicians gain from modifying their practice patterns will probably not equal the marginal cost to them in psychic terms. Thus, unless the incentives are large enough to be compelling, physicians will probably be unswayed by these systems. As the physician supply increases and maldistribution of physicians continues, however, there will be growing pressures on physicians to respond to incentive plans. Certainly for young physicians, this pressure will be strongest.

Physicians must participate in management control activities if hospitals are to have the best foundation possible for attacking the cost control problem. The failure of the past must be rectified through new methods and new intraorganizational alliances. As hospital administrators and medical directors can well testify, the failure to create a model of control that incorporates human motivation has fueled the cost crisis.

## A Cost Control Matrix

Young and Saltman attempted to associate the variables that influence hospital costs with management control.[20-22] Their work is especially good in integrating the need for cost control by administrative staff and the need for cost control by the medical staff. Furthermore, they explicitly identified the problems of integrating physicians into the management control system.

At least six major variables influence hospital costs:

1. case mix
2. number of cases
3. length of stay
4. mode of treatment
5. unit price
6. efficiency

These variables are affected by the patient and the hospital environment, the administration, and the medical staff. When all these factors are combined, the result is a matrix that hospital executives can use as a map from which they can originate strategies to improve control over hospital costs. It also can function as an assessment instrument, allowing hospital executives to determine whether they have, or do not have, control over key variables. The cost containment matrix is also an educational device that can be used to inform the board of trustees, the administrative staff, and the medical staff about the overall status of the hospital.

Finally, the matrix can be applied to DRGs. Young and Saltman suggested that DRG-based reimbursement will achieve some, but not all, of the control needed by hospitals in containing costs. The formal burden of cost control will remain on the administration. Physicians will retain enough flexibility without formal regulation to contribute voluntarily to cost control. It is their decision.

### Effect of Patients and Hospital Environment

The cost containment matrix underscores the extent to which hospitals are dependent on the patient and hospital environment for cost control. The pool of patients served by a hospital influences the case mix, and a given patient pool has unique characteristics manifested in morbidity and mortality profiles. The hospital has little opportunity to affect this profile. Similarly, the number of patients who use a hospital's services depends on the nature and disease incidence of the population. Although a high occupancy rate results in the efficient use of services, the hospital's ability to control the number of patients may be limited. Advocates of health care marketing suggest that patient use can be changed through promotional techniques, but there is no conclusive evidence that this is so.

The patient and the hospital environment also affect management's control over unit prices and efficiency. The unit price of hospital services consists of dietary wages, nursing salaries, price per unit of supplies, price per unit of radiology film, and related factor input prices. Obviously, the hospital is somewhat at the mercy of supply and demand regarding many of these input prices, but it can negotiate with suppliers, join multi-institutional purchasing groups, use its monopoly/franchise powers in smaller communities, or use other strategies to reduce unit prices. Control is generally increased more, however, by modifying the manner in which factor inputs are combined—the efficiency of using those factors. Even here, the hospital may be constrained by the external environment, because there are limitations on the extent to which the factors can be combined. For example, a nurse has a finite level of productivity; at some point, the allocation of nursing hours approaches maximum efficiency. Efforts to maximize resource use further only decrease returns.

### Effect of Administration

Hospital executives can achieve the greatest control over length of stay and the number of cases served. Although they cannot directly control how long a physician retains patients in the hospital or how many patients a physician admits to the hospital, they can limit these variables through policies that limit physician discretion. Hospital executives should set these policies in conjunction with the board of trustees and with the executive committee of the medical staff in order to avoid a confrontation with physicians.

Hospital administrators may have a diminishing ability to influence the mode of treatment. Physicians generally prefer that hospital executives make only administrative decisions and leave medical decisions to physicians. Those physicians who have this attitude are likely to resist the participation of hospital administrators in hospital cost control in relation to treatment modes. In fact, there are probably few more volatile cost containment issues than this. This would not be a good starting point for hospital executives who are interested in forming long-run, viable cost control programs; this issue is best left for the fine-tuning stage.

Hospital administrators may influence unit prices and efficiency in several ways. They may use various nursing pools to make scheduling more flexible and to reduce excessive overhead; they may participate in group purchasing plans to reduce the cost of supplies. The possibilities are as endless as the executives' imagination and capacity to translate creative ideas into practical solutions. In the same manner, they can manipulate input efficiency through the budget formulation process, the budget-monitoring process, and the establishment of accountability between budgeted and actual performance.

### Effect of Medical Staff

Physicians can control virtually every variable that influences hospital costs. They can directly affect case mix (by the patients they attract to their practice), the number of cases (by their decision to be more or less productive in their practice), the length of stay (by their judgment on retaining or discharging patients), and the mode of treatment (by their decisions about treatment regimens).

Generally, physicians have little actual control over unit prices (except their own fees). They have extraordinary control over the efficient use of hospital resources, however. They can make ancillary staff more or less productive, depending on their orders or the substitution of one type of personnel for another. To exclude physicians from a management control system could result in a noncomprehensive model that functions, but not optimally.

## LESSONS FROM HEALTH SERVICES RESEARCH

Among hospital and health services administrators, there is a growing interest in the effect of management practices on the performance of health care organizations. Recent studies have suggested that management and design variables are critical predictors of hospital efficiency and quality of care.[23-25] These results are particularly meaningful for the formation of health policy and the creation of hospital management strategies because they imply that the structure and process of health care organizations should be carefully controlled if the goals of cost containment and high-quality care are to be reached.[26,27] The focus of most health policy research continues to center on the effect of policy on outcomes, however, not on the use of policy in internal management control processes.

From a health policy perspective, prospective reimbursement should provide an incentive for health care organizations to contain costs.[28] That incentive must be internally articulated by administrators in order to achieve maximum effect. If prospective payment systems fail to stimulate creative management control mechanisms within health care organizations, such as those mentioned in this book, cost containment can be jeopardized.

Two fundamental questions remain unanswered in health services research: (1) Does prospective reimbursement encourage hospital administrators to modify their management practices? (2) Do management practices actually affect health services efficiency and quality of care? Unless research can validate the effectiveness of management control practices in cost containment, the promise of prospective payment may be eroded.

### Incentive Strategies

Many of the studies on management control practices in health care organizations do not take into account the relationship between these practices and the type of reimbursement system. Chassin, however, assessed the association between hospital cost containment and various strategies, such as those that included some form of incentive reimbursement and related the reimbursement to management practices.[29] Chassin considered six incentive reimbursement–related strategies:

1. group target ceilings
2. industrial engineering
3. department budget review
4. prospective payment by budget review
5. prospective payment by formula
6. prospective payment of total budget

Chassin categorized these cost containment strategies according to their effectiveness and efficiency in achieving the goal of cost control, as determined by a review of the pertinent health services research literature.

Although only two of the six strategies could actually be considered internal management strategies—industrial engineering and department budget review—the results presented by Chassin are at best inconclusive. Both these strategies are negatively associated with the effectiveness and the efficiency of efforts to contain hospital costs. It appears that, as hospital administrators attempt to implement more extensive industrial engineering methods or to undertake department budget reviews, the costs increase. These results suggest that hospital administrators should not concern themselves with management control. It must be remembered, however, that these conclusions were drawn from a limited number of studies that may not be universally applicable. Furthermore, the analysis of effectiveness and efficiency varied from one study to the next. Hence, caution must be used to prevent misinterpretation of the results.

Chassin's study is important, because it demonstrates the lack of research on prospective payment's impact on hospitals. The strategies of prospective payment by budget review, by formula, and by total budget have been largely overlooked in health services research—at least in regard to their effectiveness and efficiency in cost containment. More study is needed before precise conclusions regarding the intrahospital ramifications of prospective payment can be made. With Medicare's adoption of DRG-based reimbursement, it is probable that further research will soon determine whether the relationship between management practices and cost control is positive or negative.

## Costs and Management Practice in Hospitals

When Shortell, Becker, and Neuhauser studied the association between management practices and efficiency and quality of care, they did not attempt to control for the effect of the reimbursement system.[30] They focused on two primary cost variables—nonmedical support department costs and medical support department costs—in forty-two short-term, voluntary, nonteaching hospitals in Massachusetts. Their results suggested that hospitals in which the administrator is a voting member of the board of trustees and those in which a high percentage of prepared reports is sent to the board of trustees are more likely to have lower nonmedical support department costs. Shortell, Becker, and Neuhauser attributed this to the visibility of the consequences of administrative practice (i.e., the board will be cognizant of good or bad managerial performance).

In the nonmedical support department cost analysis, other significant variables were also noted. The percentage of reports prepared, as well as the percentage of operating statistics known by the administrator, was associated with reduced costs. These results may indicate that it is not the process (i.e., report preparation or performance analysis) that distinguishes management control practices; it is the manner in which those practices are implemented.

In examining medical support department costs for the forty-two hospitals, Shortell, Becker, and Neuhauser found that costs increase when key administrative personnel, such as the chief of staff, lack knowledge about basic operating statistics. It appears that, in order to contain costs, administrators must have a basic knowledge about operating statistics. Again, Shortell, Becker, and Neuhauser attributed this result to the visibility of consequence.

Medical support department costs decreased when the number of regularly scheduled meetings involving personnel from the radiology, nursing, and laboratory departments was increased. This suggests that more coordination leads to lower costs, an intuitively understandable result. Higher management coordination produces a more efficient work process, which is ultimately distilled in lower costs.

In order to determine the impact of management practices on hospital length of stay, Becker, Shortell, and Neuhauser divided length of stay into average (total) length of stay, Medicare length of stay, and Medicare preoperative length of stay. They found that the total length of stay was shorter when hospital administrators could compare their hospital's performance to that of other hospitals in the community. Similarly, the average length of stay decreased when work was more extensively specified for medical support department heads. This work specification should include definite goals of the hospital. These proxy measures of management control practices suggest that average length of stay can be directly affected by the control implemented.

The implications of this study for management control under DRG-based reimbursement are interesting, given the prediction that many hospitals will decrease the average length of stay to improve financial returns from a given DRG reimbursement rate. It appears that hospitals should consider expanding management control practices of this nature if they want to reduce the average length of stay. However, there may be better methods that Becker, Shortell, and Neuhauser did not analyze (e.g., incentives for physicians who maintain a low average length of stay).

## Implications from Nursing Homes

The applicability of prospective payment to long-term care expenditures is receiving more and more attention. There is a considerable need for additional evaluation studies of prospective rate reimbursement in nursing homes, however, since Medicaid expenditures for long-term care will rise in direct proportion to the aging of the national population. Unless nursing home expenditures are more firmly controlled (e.g., through more efficient reimbursement systems or through the introduction of noninstitutional alternatives to long-term care), the next several decades may witness a crisis in expenditures for long-term care analogous to that for hospital care.

We have undertaken a study to determine whether there is any difference between the internal management control practices of long-term care facilities that are prospectively reimbursed and those of facilities that are not prospectively reimbursed. The study included nursing homes in Alabama, California, and Washington (state). At the time of the study, Alabama facilities were reimbursed on an inclusive per diem rate. The California facilities were reimbursed on a modified per diem rate; the size (i.e., number of beds) and patient mix (i.e., percentage of Medicaid patients) determined in which of three rate categories a nursing home could be placed for reimbursement purposes. Finally, Washington used a prospective rate reimbursement system based on a cost profile, adjusted for industry averages, for each nursing home.

Compared with the per diem rates, prospective payment seems likely to provide increasing incentives for good administrative practices. We anticipate better budgeting, planning, and decision making. Since the facilities are at financial risk, they have an incentive to implement management practices designed to contain costs. The intensity of care (i.e., the number of skilled nursing hours per patient day) may be maximized, because it may generate higher legitimate costs for nursing services. With higher legitimate nursing costs, the per diem reimbursement rate therefore is also higher. In this manner, a health care organization might be able to create short-run slack in the budget. The role of profits is uncertain. It has been predicted that prospective payment will decrease incentives for profits, since the intention of most prospective payment systems is to limit public health expenditures.

Per diem rate reimbursement systems do not provide incentives for good administrative practice that are *comparable* to the incentives associated with prospective payment systems. While incentives under prospective payment are to hold down costs, incentives under per diem reimbursement favor pursuit of profits. Usually, a "reasonable" return on investment is targeted as the profit goal. There may be incentives to minimize intensity of care in order to attain a greater operating margin.

For nursing homes, regulations are oriented mainly toward ensuring standards of care for Medicaid patients. Thus, nursing homes with a high percentage of Medicaid patients are likely to have more management controls (in view of government regulations and their enforcement by state agencies) than do nursing homes with a low percentage of Medicaid patients (i.e., many private pay patients). Therefore, the percentage of Medicaid patients can be used as a control variable. We divided each sample for each state into two portions—those with a high percentage of Medicaid patients and those with a low percentage. Since it is impossible to adjust totally for differences across the three states, this bifurcation permits an understanding of the impact of regulation on the association between reimbursement system and internal management practices.

The study was conducted among 65 Alabama, 43 California, and 70 Washington skilled nursing facilities. Under each reimbursement system, three different dependent variables were analyzed: (1) total cost per patient day, (2) profit per patient day, and (3) intensity of care per patient day. (In the Alabama facilities, however, no profit data were obtainable.) Total cost and profit per patient day are standard measures of economic efficiency. Profit per patient day was calculated from the difference between total income per patient day and total costs per patient day. The intensity of care per patient day was determined from the number of skilled nursing hours per patient day reported to the state health agencies.

The major independent variable, internal management control practices, is expected to be negatively related to costs and intensity of care, and positively related to profit. If a reimbursement system provides an incentive for effective management control practices, those nursing homes with greater control practices should also be those with higher profits, lower costs, and a higher intensity of care.

Although there were no significant variables entered in the Washington sample for costs, the profit and skilled nursing hours regressions associated with a high percentage of Medicaid patients both indicate that management practices represent statistically significant ($p < .01$) predictors (Table 7–2). Higher profits and a lower intensity of care were found in Washington nursing homes that actively implement management control practices.

---

**Table 7–2** Association of Management Control and Performance in Nursing Homes

| | Statistically Significant Predictors per State | | |
| --- | --- | --- | --- |
| | Alabama | California | Washington |
| High Medicaid patient payer mix Dependent variables | | | |
| Cost | None | YEARAD (+) | None |
| Profit | No data | None | MGT (+) |
| Skilled Nursing Hours | MGT (−) | TBEDS (+) YEARAD (+) | MGT (−) |
| Low Medicaid patient payer mix Dependent variables | | | |
| Cost | None | None | YEARAD (−) |
| Profit | No data | None | None |
| Skilled Nursing Hours | TBEDS (−) | OCC (−) | None |

---

*Key:* MGT = management control practices
YEARAD = years in administration for the top administrator
TBEDS = total bed size
OCC = occupancy
+ = positive association
− = negative association

Management practices represented a statistically significant predictor of intensity of care for the Alabama sample, but there were no other statistically relevant results for Alabama. The California sample did not indicate any significant associations for management control activities. Furthermore, no significant variables were found for profit in the California group. The experience of the administrator in the nursing home field was a statistically significant predictor for both costs and intensity of care in the California facilities, however. Administrators with little experience were associated with higher costs and lower intensity of care in the California nursing homes. Finally, a high number of total beds was associated with high intensity of care nursing homes in California.

Overall, the multiple regressions in Table 7–2 suggest that management control practices are most closely associated with profit and intensity of care for Washington state nursing homes (under prospective reimbursement) and with intensity of care for Alabama nursing homes (under an inclusive per diem rate). Thus, the predicted relationships are partially supported.

Clearly, there was a much greater prevalence of nonsignificant predictors in the statistical analyses of facilities with a low percentage of Medicaid patients. This was especially true for management control practices, since this variable was not a statistically significant predictor of the dependent variables. Each state had at least one regression in which significant results were attained, yet there was no consistent pattern among the statistically significant independent variables.

Management control practices were associated with higher profit and lower intensity of care in nursing homes that had a high percentage of Medicaid patients and were reimbursed through a prospective system. Management control practices were also associated with a lower intensity of care in one group of facilities under the per diem reimbursement system (Alabama). There was no evidence that management control practices explain variance in nursing home performance (i.e., cost, profit, or skilled nursing hours) in the sample of nursing homes with a low percentage of Medicaid patients. It is possible, therefore, that prospective rate reimbursement does provide an additional incentive for efficient operations in health care facilities.

## Conclusions for Hospital Management

There is growing evidence that suggests that management control practices may be associated with lower costs in health care facilities. These preliminary findings are the result of studies which have generally omitted the form of reimbursement as a critical research variable. Thus, caution must be used in extrapolating from these studies to specific management practices. Additional research needs to be completed that tests for cogency of the associations noted for prospective payment. For the present, DRGs will add a new challenge to hospital administration that further tests the capacity of administrators to achieve cost control.

**NOTES**

1. William L. Dowling, "Prospective Rate Setting: Concept and Practice," in *Managing the Finances of Health Care Organizations,* ed. G.E. Bisbee and R.A. Vraciu (Ann Arbor: Health Administration Press, 1980).

2. David W. Young and Richard B. Saltman, "Prospective Reimbursement and the Hospital Power Equilibrium: A Matrix-Based Management Control System," *Inquiry* 20 (1983):20–33.

3. Selwyn W. Becker, Stephen M. Shortell, and Duncan Neuhauser, "Management Practices and Hospital Length of Stay," *Inquiry* 17 (1980):318–330.

4. Frank A. Sloan and Bruce Steinwald, "Effects of Regulation on Hospital Costs and Use," *Journal of Law and Economics* 23 (1980):81–109.

5. Craig Coelen and Daniel Sullivan, "An Analysis of the Effects of Prospective Reimbursement Programs on Hospital Expenditures," *Health Care Financing Review* 5 (1981):1–40.

6. Stephen M. Shortell, Selwyn W. Becker, and Duncan Neuhauser, "The Effects of Management Practices on Hospital Efficiency and Quality of Care," in *Organizational Research in Hospitals,* ed. Stephen M. Shortell and Montague Brown (Chicago: Inquiry, 1976).

7. Howard L. Smith, Myron D. Fottler, and Borje O. Saxberg, "Cost Containment in Health Care: A Model for Management Research," *Academy of Management Review* 6 (1981):397–407.

8. Beaufort B. Longest, *Management Practices for the Health Care Professional* (Reston, Va.: Reston Publishing, 1980).

9. Howard L. Smith, David J. Ottensmeyer, and Derick P. Pasternak, "Physician Incentive Compensation in Group Practice: A Review with Suggestions for Improvement," *Health Care Management Review* 9 (1984):41–49.

10. Regina E. Herzlinger and Gordon T. Moore, "Management Control Systems in Health Care," *Medical Care* 11 (1973):416–428.

11. Lois Meyers and Steven Schroeder, "Physician Use of Services for the Hospitalized Patient: A Review with Implications for Cost Containment," *Milbank Memorial Fund Quarterly* 59 (1981):41.

12. John M. Eisenberg, "An Educational Program to Modify Laboratory Use by House Staff," *Journal of Medical Education* 52 (1977):578.

13. Regina E. Herzlinger, "Can We Control Health Care Costs?" *Harvard Business Review* 56 (1978): 102–116.

14. Herzlinger and Moore, "Management Control Systems in Health Care."

15. William O. Cleverly and Robert P. Mullen, "Management Incentive Systems and Economic Performance in Health Care Organizations," *Health Care Management Review* 7 (1982):7–14.

16. Howard L. Smith and Myron D. Fottler, "Costs and Cost Containment in Nursing Homes," *Health Services Research* 16 (1981):17–41.

17. Carol McCarthy, "Incentive Reimbursement As an Impetus to Cost Containment," *Inquiry* 12 (1975):320–329.

18. Cleverly and Mullen, "Management Incentive Systems and Economic Performance."

19. Smith, Ottensmeyer, and Pasternak, "Physician Incentive Compensation in Group Practice."

20. David W. Young and Richard B. Saltman, "Medical Practice, Case Mix, and Cost Containment," *Journal of the American Medical Association* #247 (1982):801–804.

21. Young and Saltman, "Prospective Reimbursement and the Hospital Power Equilibrium."

22. David W. Young and Richard B. Saltman, "Preventive Medicine for Hospital Costs," *Harvard Business Review* 61 (1983):126–133.

23. Edward V. Morse, Gerald Gordon, and Michael Moch, "Hospital Costs and Quality of Care: An Organizational Perspective," *MMFQ* 52 (1974):315–345.

24. W. Richard Scott, Ann Barry Flood, and Wayne Ewy, "Organizational Determinants of Services, Quality and Cost of Care in Hospitals," *Milbank Memorial Fund Quarterly* 57 (1979):234–257.

25. Becker, Shortell, and Neuhauser, "Management Practices and Hospital Length of Stay."

26. Avedis Donabedian, "Evaluating the Quality of Medical Care," *Milbank Memorial Fund Quarterly* 44 (1966):166—206.

27. Duncan Neuhauser and Ronald Anderson, "Structural-Comparative Studies of Hospitals," in *Organizational Research on Health Institutions*, ed. Basil S. Georgopoulos (Ann Arbor, Mich.: University of Michigan, 1972).

28. Young and Saltman, "Prospective Reimbursement and the Hospital Power Equilibrium."

29. Mark R. Chassin, "The Containment of Hospital Costs: A Strategic Assessment," *Medical Care* 16 (1978, supplement):46–55.

30. Shortell, Becker, and Neuhauser, "The Effects of Management Practices on Hospital Efficiency and Quality of Care."

# Chapter 8

# Organizing for DRGs

Under the prospective payment system, hospital managers and personnel must cope with restraints that are very different from those to which they are accustomed. If those hospitals that depend on Medicare as a primary source of income are to survive under the system, they must make rapid adjustments in organizing for reimbursement based on diagnosis-related groups (DRGs) and creating mechanisms to control resource use. All hospital managers must develop strategies to meet the challenge, anticipating the needs of the hospital and directing its diverse elements in a way that ensures economic and organizational stability.

## ORGANIZATIONAL CHANGE

In adopting their institution to a prospective payment system, hospital managers must change the organizational attitudes toward resource usage that developed under the previous retrospective payment system. Thus, it will be necessary to change the consumption habits fostered under the ''cost plus'' pricing method by promoting cost containment, efficient management, and appropriate utilization of resources. Hospital managers must start with their own attitudes and develop habits designed to alter previously dominant behavior. The advent of change in the hospital must be managed carefully. Yet, prospective payment offers only two alternatives: (1) to operate at costs below those determined by DRG rates and remain solvent, or (2) to allow overall costs to rise above those determined by DRG rates, incur a loss, and threaten the institution with bankruptcy.

The most important element in the implementation of changes is to encourage interdepartmental and multidisciplinary communication in order to identify potential areas for cost savings and increased efficiency. This requires the creation of an internal managerial climate and structure that fosters efficiency.

Top management must insist that all staff members learn to read the appropriate computerized reports concerning costs and resource usage. Obviously, this can occur only if effective management information systems exist and this information is provided to the responsible managers. Only top management can decide to develop and/or purchase the sophisticated managerial information systems needed, but DRG information must be available at all organizational levels.

Several types of organization may be appropriate as hospitals attempt to adapt to the prospective payment system: the appointment of a task force to implement the new system, appointment of a DRG coordinator, or alternate organizational structures. All of these organizational structures require the development and offering of various staff education programs.

## DRG TASK FORCE

Responding to DRG-based reimbursement demands coordinated effort from every level of the hospital. The task force, which is commonly and effectively used for problem solving in business and government, can be employed by hospitals as well for managing prospective reimbursement. The sweeping changes required by prospective payment become apparent to all personnel with the appointment of this task force. Therefore, one of the first organizational changes should be the appointment of a DRG task force or committee in order to show that the organization is serious about making the changes necessary to operate under prospective reimbursement.

A DRG task force composed of department heads from various hospital operations organized under the chief financial officer is one useful model. The task force would be responsible for developing and implementing the hospital's organizational strategy toward prospective payment.[1] Membership on the task force is essential for certain departments, such as the finance department, the medical records department, accounting or patient billing, utilization review, the data-processing department, nursing, and administration.[2] By working together as a team, representatives of these departments must ensure that the organization will operate effectively and efficiently under prospective reimbursement.

Obviously, members of the task force must become "in-house" experts on DRGs by familiarizing themselves with the guidelines for prospective reimbursement available in the *Federal Register* and with the recommendations now being widely distributed in the health services literature.[3] Understanding the system will help the representatives of the various departments to assess the effects of the new system on their respective departments and to determine the best approach to management. More important, the members can formulate changes that all departments must implement in unison by setting and coordinating departmental goals within an overall organizational plan for managing DRGs.

A member of the executive management team who is respected, action-oriented, and articulate should chair the task force.[4] Without this type of visible authority, it may be difficult to coordinate the diverse organizational elements for consensus action; the result will be organizational inertia and inability to meet the requirements of the new system.

The chief financial officer may be responsible for heading the task force, establishing work deadlines, and maintaining a line of communication between the task force, the administration, and the medical staff.[5] He or she needs a full commitment of time, resources, and personnel to ensure successful completion of the job. Assessment of the overall impact of DRGs on the hospital is the chief financial officer's basic objective. This assessment is made by using historical data from many different sources to project hospital revenues and costs under DRGs.

Obviously, the role of the medical records department will be significantly enlarged under prospective reimbursement. The medical records director must adapt the medical record system to increase the accuracy and completeness of information for billing Medicare. Hospitals will not be reimbursed by Medicare for the care provided to patients whose medical records are incomplete; therefore, coding methods must be improved to avoid slowed payment and increase profits.[6] A closer association must be developed between medical records, data processing, and the medical staff in order to integrate clinical data with the financial data necessary for DRG-based reimbursement.[7] The importance of developing a single *integrated* data base cannot be overemphasized.

New information systems for DRGs are the forte of the data processing manager. He or she must determine the computer hardware and software needed by the hospital for DRG-based reimbursement. The data processing manager coordinates the collection of clinical data from the patient's admission until discharge.[8] These data are used to place the illness in its proper DRG. The managerial implications of linking these data to costs for each service provided in each DRG are enormous if product-oriented reports result. Operational and productivity information should be calculated on the basis of the hospital's case mix. This permits more efficient management by proper staffing and scheduling according to patient need.

The utilization review director monitors physician and departmental DRG profiles of resource consumption. This control system identifies the centers within the organization that generate revenues and those that are responsible for costs. Measures can then be taken to address and control the problem areas.

The accounting manager ensures that financial records are accurate and monitors the effects of DRG-based reimbursement on the hospital's financial standing.[9] Standard cost accounting techniques are useful in the control of various costs in hospital operations. The accounting manager also assists the financial officer in making future projections of costs and revenue. The functions of various task force members in one hospital are shown in Table 8–1.

8888888

8888

**Table 8–1** Tasks of Prospective Payment Implementation Task Force, Columbus-Cuneo-Cabrini Medical Center, Chicago

| Member | Primary Tasks | Secondary Tasks |
|---|---|---|
| Vice-president, finance | Assess PPS's impact on bottom line, communicate with COOs, act as task force facilitator | |
| Director, medical records | Organize DRG information systems, review preadmission testing process to shift cost to outpatient, since Medicare provides 100 percent reimbursement for such tests | Organize education programs |
| Director, utilization review | Analyze potential utilization problems, rank physicians and DRGs by profitability | Identify outliers |
| Director, reimbursement | Analyze cash flow effects, maximize prospective payment by cost allocation among three hospitals, estimate PPS's effect on 1984 budgets | Maintain constant communication with Medicare intermediary |
| Controller | Institute billing changes, prepare financial statements | Organize patient logs |
| Director, data processing | Organize DRG information systems, patient logs, and billing systems | |
| Cost accounting manager | Identify the true cost of providing care, treatment, and procedures using a more precise method than Medicare cost-to-charge ratios | Assess units that are excluded from PPS/capital costs and pass-throughs |
| Director, patient care services | Organize education programs | Teach departments, physicians who purchase from outside vendors—and the vendors—to make sure that purchasing patterns do not violate the new regulations |

*Note:* PPS, prospective payment system; COO, chief operating officer

*Source:* Reprinted from Richard J. Annis, "Task Force, Staff Education, Ease Transition to Prospective Payment," *Hospital Progress* 65 (February 1984):52. Used with permission from the Catholic Health Association of the United States, St. Louis, Mo.

The task force method allows an organization to employ its top personnel in solving a problem. In the short run, the task force method is the best response for organizing the institution's management of prospective reimbursement. It is not a long-run solution to DRG-posed problems, however. Some hospitals may use the task force throughout the three-year implementation period; others may prefer to use the task force to develop the initial strategy for managing DRGs and to develop long-term strategies through their board of directors. In other cases, the task force may be converted into a permanent committee with permanent authority to implement significant changes.

The important goal is to involve individuals in all organizational levels and functions in the planning process to ensure a coordinated response to prospective payment. In addition, a permanent administrative structure must be developed to manage the hospital under the new system.

## STAFF EDUCATION

### General

All hospitals must decide at the outset how best to educate their staff about DRGs, since the effectiveness of staff education determines the smoothness of the transition from retrospective to prospective Medicare reimbursement. Some hospitals employ large educational assemblies of all hospital personnel for training purposes, but this may be logistically infeasible. It may be more appropriate to design educational seminars targeted at the effects of DRGs on each particular department. For example, seminars for nurses and nursing administrators could emphasize productivity, cost control, reduction of unnecessary patient stays, and decreased use of ancillary services.[10] Educational sessions for hospital trustees should concentrate on long-range strategic planning under prospective reimbursement, impact of DRGs on operations, development of new product lines, and key features of reimbursement under DRGs.[11]

Organization of these seminars and/or workshops should be coordinated by departmental supervisors and/or the DRG coordinator. The finance and accounting department should provide specific financial data for each department and the effect of prospective reimbursement on each department's financial operations. These data allow departmental personnel to compare and contrast their operations under retrospective reimbursement with those under prospective reimbursement.

At these seminars, various training media permit maximum exposure during a short allotted time. The hospital should develop a comprehensive training manual that employees can use at their educational sessions. Later, employees can refer to the manual when questions arise about their own jobs. These materials can be developed in-house or can be purchased from publishing houses. Department-specific literature to supplement this material may also be useful. Many organizations choose video presentations for training. Although the combination of audio and video clarifies the material presented, the cost may exceed budgetary limitations. Less expensive alternatives are slide presentations, flip charts, and print media. Internal hospital media, such as newsletters, should be used to keep all personnel up-to-date on changes in the prospective payment system as they occur and on the progress of hospital operations in the transition to DRG-based reimbursement.

The ultimate goal of staff education is to inform all hospital personnel of the risks that the organization faces under DRG-based reimbursement. Personnel must understand that the economic health and viability of the institution that provides their jobs relies on a coordinated effort to control costs and to manage resources efficiently. This can be accomplished only by incorporating staff into the planning of hospital policy. Given the opportunity to participate in policy formulation, develop personal and departmental goals, and provide feedback on the results, most employees respond positively to the challenge. Management should encourage initiative in creating innovative solutions to any problems arising under prospective reimbursement. For example, labor-management cooperation in unionized hospitals can ease the transition of hospital operations to DRG-based reimbursement.

## Physician Education

One of the major tasks for hospital administrators in the management of DRG-based reimbursement is to reorient physician practice patterns toward the efficient, cost-effective consumption of hospital resources. Physicians must reexamine the decision-making process involved in the provision of patient services (see Chapter 11). Since a financial risk is associated with the diagnosis and treatment of each case, a physician who misdiagnoses a condition, overuses ancillary services, allows the patient to remain in the hospital too long, or makes any number of clinical mistakes that increase costs may cause the hospital to run a deficit on the reimbursement for that particular DRG.

One problem inherent to prospective payment is that there are no built-in incentives in the system to encourage physicians to control clinical consumption patterns. It is assumed that hospital administrators exercise considerable managerial control over the medical staff. This is generally not the case, however.[12] Therefore, the successful operation of hospitals under DRG-based reimbursement must be a joint venture of the management and the medical staff. Both groups must be dedicated and willing to share the risk and responsibility of managing DRGs effectively.[13] The difficulty arises when physicians object to careful scrutiny and criticism of medical practice patterns that were considered reasonable under the old retrospective reimbursement system.

The medical staff must understand clearly that physicians unable to function within DRG standards must modify their practices. The hospital manager and medical staff director (or chief of staff) must confront the individual physician and receive assurances that the necessary changes will be made. Therefore, it is essential to have accurate, significant, and verifiable data on utilization.

The hospital is an entity basically designed for physicians to provide medical care to their patients. All other functions support the provision of these medical services. The hospital manager is responsible for maintaining the hospital and its facilities, however, and one of the most difficult but necessary tasks faced by the hospital manager is to develop a consensus with the medical staff concerning organization, policies, and procedures required to operate under the constraints of prospective reimbursement. Communication is the key. A professional working relationship between the medical staff and management can achieve both high-quality health care and economic viability, even under the restriction of DRG-based reimbursement. Each party must understand the role it plays in reaching these goals.

## THE DRG COORDINATOR

The creation of a management function to oversee the three-year transition period during which the Medicare program is being implemented is a high priority for hospital managers. Accordingly, many hospitals have created a staff position (i.e., DRG coordinator) or even an entirely new department to coordinate hospital changes under DRG-based reimbursement.

A DRG coordinator could be drawn from any one of several hospital departments, including finance, data processing, or medical records. Smaller hospitals may designate a member of one of these departments to serve as a coordinator on a part-time basis or as a resident expert on DRGs. The size and needs of the hospital determine the scope of the position. Because the designated DRG coordinator plays a major role in hospital operations, at least for the first three years of DRG-based reimbursement, he or she must have the managerial skill to integrate DRGs into the existing management system. Later, he or she must slowly reorient hospital operations in order to incorporate strategic changes and policy changes at the operational (i.e., departmental) level.

### Role of the DRG Coordinator

The DRG coordinator's role in assisting hospital managers varies from hospital to hospital. In some hospitals, the DRG coordinator may simply monitor DRG information and guidelines to ensure a case-by-case medical record compilation.[14] In other hospitals, the DRG coordinator has a very broad role, being responsible for tasks such as developing training seminars and workshops, preparing educational literature, acting as an intermediary between management and medical staff, developing a resource utilization review system based on DRGs, and corresponding with the Medicare agencies.

The DRG coordinator participates in the education of the hospital staff and assists in creating educational literature (e.g., brochures for patients, employee training manuals, press releases for community media, video presentations) that describes DRGs and prospective payment in terms understandable to the layman. Working with various department heads, the DRG coordinator develops programs for seminars targeted at the needs of the particular hospital department. Continuing education and information about changes in the prospective payment system as affected by the federal government can be provided to hospital personnel by mailings or through the hospital newsletter.

The DRG coordinator often serves as an ombudsman when DRG problems arise within the hospital. He or she coordinates the interaction and communication among those departments that have the most important functions under the new system (i.e., medical records, finance, and the medical staff). The DRG coordinator also monitors DRG-pertinent hospital interrelationships and political developments during the transition period. These activities should help the hospital to avoid potential conflicts and obstacles to achievement of organizational goals.

Finally, the DRG coordinator can serve a crucial financial interface role with those activities taking place internally and externally to identify problems (real and potential), examine the financial impact, and communicate this information to departments. He or she monitors new reports on Medicare patients to keep hospital executives up-to-date on the fiscal impact of DRGs on the hospital.

## Data Gathering and Analysis

One of the DRG coordinator's most important tasks is to integrate clinical and financial data for data processing, medical records, billing, and utilization review. The hospital must have modern management information systems in order to ensure its survival under DRG-based reimbursement. Accuracy and speed of information flow from patient admission to billing are primary goals.

The DRG coordinator should help to modify the data processing capabilities of the hospital so that costs per case can be monitored as patients move through the system. The computer hardware and software industry has developed a host of products that can be used in gathering, processing, and analyzing financial and clinical information under DRG-based reimbursement.[15] These systems are only as good as the data entered into them, however. They require accurate clinical information from line personnel, accurate coding by medical records staff, and quality analysis by data processing staff.

New systems and procedures to enhance the quality of data must be developed.[16] Records are classified according to DRG, age, sex, principal diagnosis, secondary diagnosis, surgical procedures, and other information coded by the *International Classification of Diseases, 9th Revision, Clinical Modification* (ICD–9–CM) codes for DRGs.[17] Because errors in recording this clinical information can result in reimbursement delays or loss,[18] the DRG coordinator should establish a review system to monitor the accuracy and completeness of medical records before they are submitted for reimbursement.

The DRG coordinator uses case data from these medical records to calculate the cost standards used in the physician, nursing, and ancillary services utilization review. Further analysis of these records reveals the actual costs that the hospital incurs per DRG, the physician practice patterns under these DRGs, and the resources consumed per DRG. Hospital administrators use this information to identify problem areas, take corrective action, and determine which DRGs are most profitable.

Every hospital experiences conflict if or when the status quo is altered. Easing the transition to DRG-based reimbursement and managing the conflict associated with it fall into the hands of the DRG coordinator, department heads, and hospital administrators. The conversion from a health care strategy based on a consumer orientation to one with a product orientation will be a difficult transition for hospitals. A DRG coordinator can facilitate the process by helping hospital personnel to understand what changes can be expected and why these changes are required.

## ALTERNATE ORGANIZATIONAL STRUCTURES

Instead of establishing an autonomous position for a DRG coordinator, some hospitals may prefer to manage the transition to DRG-based reimbursement by establishing a separate department or a new position as assistant to the top administrator. Large hospitals, teaching hospitals, and hospitals heavily dependent on Medicare patients may benefit from a departmental arrangement in which personnel are appropriated from the departments heavily involved in the DRG reimbursement process, such as the finance, medical records, data processing, accounting, and patient care services departments. This form of organization has the advantage of allowing a representative of each department affected to participate in the formulation of DRG policy for the hospital. In addition, the needs of each department can be addressed by the DRG department member taken from that area of the operation. Thus, a more comprehensive and effective policy could result.

In the early stages of the planning process, the DRG department can be organized under the guidance of the DRG task force, which is usually composed of the heads of the same departments from which personnel for the DRG department are chosen. The DRG department then slowly assumes the burden of the task force planning function, while developing many of the programs that otherwise would fall to a DRG coordinator. Each member interacts directly with his or her respective department during the implementation of DRG control mechanisms. After the hospital has achieved a complete transition to DRG-based reimbursement, the DRG department may be disbanded and replaced by a DRG coordinator.

The departmental approach requires a sizable commitment of money, time, and resources by the hospital administration. Therefore, some type of cost-benefit analysis should be conducted prior to the adoption of this approach. Small and/or rural hospitals, particularly those in which the administration exercises great unilateral control over hospital operations, may find it preferable to designate an assistant to the top administrator to coordinate DRG policy. This approach requires a much smaller commitment of human and economic resources.

The hospital administrator designates a member of his or her staff or employs a new assistant administrator to organize the hospital's transition to DRG-based reimbursement. The chief financial officer, an administrator from the finance department, or (in smaller hospitals) an assistant administrator responsible for monitoring hospital finances may be candidates for the job. This approach to DRGs requires greater caution than do other approaches. Prospective reimbursement necessitates organizationwide changes, and participative management during the transition improves the effectiveness of these changes. Unilateral decision making from the top administration may create conflict and hostility toward organizational goals at the department and medical staff levels. In order to avoid these problems, the assistant to the administrator must encourage feedback and compromise from hospital personnel. A team approach ensures consensus agreement and helps every participant to recognize that the hospital's future depends on the appropriate responses to DRGs at every level in the organization.

---

NOTES

1. Cynthia Wallace, "Hospitals Getting Ready for DRG's," *Modern Healthcare* 13 (December 1983): 23.

2. Richard J. Annis, "Task Force, Staff Education, Ease Transition to Prospective Payment," *Hospital Progress* 65 (February 1984): 51.

3. Ibid.

4. Ibid.

5. Annis, "Task Force, Staff Education," 52.

6. Ibid.

7. Michael Nathanson, "Medical Records' New Financial Role Dramatically Shifts Hospital Priorities," *Modern Healthcare* 13 (April 1983): 50.

8. Annis, "Task Force, Staff Education," 74.

9. Franklin A. Schaffer, "Gearing Up for DRG's: Management Strategies," *Nursing and Health Care* 5 (February 1984): 95.

10. Sallie M. Olsen, "The Challenge of Prospective Pricing: Work Smarter," *The Journal of Nursing Administration* 14 (April 1984): 22.

11. Annis, "Task Force, Staff Education," 50.

12. Wallace, "Hospitals Getting Ready for DRG's," 28.

13. John G. Nackel, P. Douglas Powell, and Michael Goran, "Case-Mix Management: Issues and Strategies," *Hospital and Health Services Administration* 29 (January/February 1984): 13.

14. Wallace, "Hospitals Getting Ready for DRG's," 23.

15. Richard F. Averill, Michael J. Kauson, David A. Sparrow, and Thomas R. Owens, "How Hospital Managers Should Respond to PPS," *Healthcare Financial Management* 4 (March 1984): 72.

16. Ibid.

17. Ibid.

18. Ibid., 76.

# Chapter 9

# Tactical Factors: Medical Records and Billing

Few management factors require greater accuracy under a system of prospective reimbursement based on diagnosis-related groups (DRGs) than do medical records and billing. Medical records department personnel must be precise in record keeping to ensure that the hospital receives the correct level of reimbursement. Then, the billing or patient account department must receive from the medical records department the correct charge for distribution to third party reimbursers and to the patient. Although these tasks are simple in concept, they are often difficult to implement accurately because of poorly conceived management information systems and the high volume of patient accounts that must be processed. Accuracy in medical record keeping and in patient billing is the cornerstone for the meaningful management of DRGs and prospective payment, however. The precise changes that must occur in the medical records department and the billing office are complex. Hospitals must move from strategically defining plans for managing DRGs to actually deploying resources in order to implement the plans.

## PARAMETERS OF PATIENT CLASSIFICATION

DRGs will affect cost containment and quality assurance. This is a strategic concept that forms a basis from which specific plans and decisions can be made within the hospital. Until hospitals have clearly underscored the multidimensionality of DRGs, the importance of collaborative interfaces among all medical and nonmedical departments, and the need to manage DRGs within a common frame of reference, it is unlikely that the resulting plans and performance of the various departments will attain anything but mediocrity.

Burik and Nackel argued that DRGs should be viewed mainly as a patient classification system around which hospitals structure their cost containment and quality assurance efforts.[1] This argument is compelling, because it suggests that strategic and operational plans within hospitals are dependent on the manner in which patients are classified. Yet, patient classification is subject to extensive interpretation. For example, the complexity of patient care—and the resulting patient mix—is defined by the severity of illness, its prognosis, the difficulty of treatment, the pressure for timely treatment, and the level of resources invested in treating a patient.[2]

Although prospective payment systems will vary from state to state, patient classification systems are likely to echo DRGs. According to Grimaldi and Micheletti, the main parameters of patient classification under DRGs are

1. operating room procedure
2. principal diagnosis
3. age of patient admission
4. sex of patient
5. complication or co-morbidity
6. secondary diagnoses[3]

When a patient undergoes an operating room procedure for kidney or urinary tract disease, for example, the principal diagnosis, patient age, patient sex, development of any complications, and secondary diagnosis parameters function as classification criteria (Figure 9–1). The operating room procedure eventually leads to the patient's classification in one of DRGs 302 to 315. For a patient who does not require an operating room or surgical procedure, the principal diagnosis could be either renal failure, a neoplasm, infection, stone, signs and symptoms, urethral stricture, or other disease. This patient is assigned to one of DRGs 316 to 333 (Figure 9–2).

Although there are significant problems in determining the precise DRG classification for each patient, this approach is not a radically different method of classifying patients at the point of diagnosis. The major difference between the International Classification of Diseases and the hospital adaptation is in the grouping of patients according to six classification parameters. A procedure known as AUTOGRP (i.e., automatic grouping system) may be used to file diseases and diagnoses into relatively homogeneous categories.[4,5] This statistical grouping has thus been tempered by the input of clinical judgment to create DRGs that are medically meaningful.

For hospital executives, the practical significance of the classification method is that it requires them to create a system of quality control. Reliable information must be gathered for strategic plans and decisions pertaining to institutional operations. The director of the medical records department must share in this process of control over patient classification. Although these executives cannot exer-

**Figure 9–1** Diseases and Disorders of the Kidney and Urinary Tract for Surgical Procedure

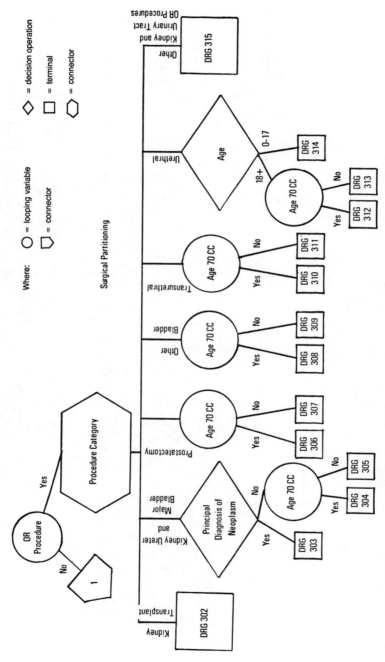

*Source:* Reprinted from *DRGs: A Practitioner's Guide* by Paul L. Grimaldi and Julie A. Micheletti with permission of Pluribus Press, Inc., 160 E. Illinois Street, Chicago, IL 60611.

**Figure 9–2** Diseases and Disorders of the Kidney and Urinary Tract without a Qualifying Surgical Procedure

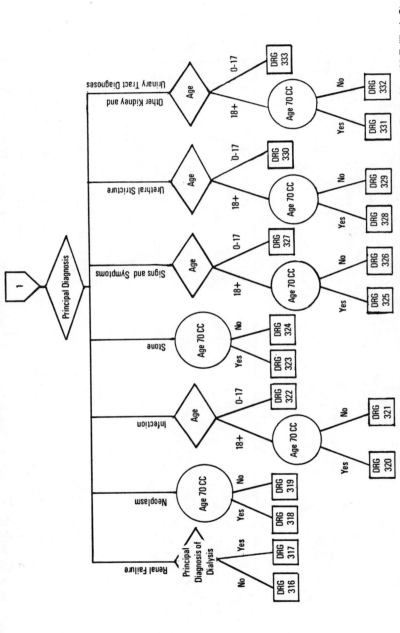

*Source:* Reprinted from *DRGs: A Practitioner's Guide* by Paul L. Grimaldi and Julie A. Micheletti with permission of Pluribus Press, Inc., 160 E. Illinois Street, Chicago, IL. 60611.

cise influence over patient groupings—the parameters are already incorporated within the principal diagnosis methodology—they can attend to the operational systems under which patient assignments are made and coded within the information system of the hospital.

Patient classification has substantial implications for the billing office or patient accounts department as well. The accuracy of bills sent from the hospital must be controlled in order to maximize reimbursement. Hospital executives must be alert to events within the billing and medical records departments. They must define the methods by which the work of each department is integrated to produce accurate and timely results. Hospital executives must also manage the information flowing from these departments. The revenue and cost data, with the patient case mix data, can affect the current and planned performance of the hospital.

Business office managers or department supervisors for patient accounts must be cognizant of the ramifications of DRGs in managing the processes of their departments. The process used to complete a medical record to ensure maximum reimbursement involves three key stages in the operations of the medical records and billing departments (Figure 9–3):

1. Patient charts are completed in the clinical or nursing unit.
2. Patient charts are forwarded to the medical records department for coding according to the DRG format.
3. Patient charts are forwarded to the billing department for preparation in submitting payment.

Each of these stages carries important strategic management implications.

## STRATEGIC MANAGEMENT OF MEDICAL RECORDS

The medical records department's role is amplified the moment a patient is admitted to the hospital. The medical record not only is the main source from which data are gathered for reimbursement purposes, but also establishes a basis from which other decisions and plans can be developed in the hospital. Medical records have always been important as a source of information regarding services provided and sources of funds, but under DRG-based reimbursement and other prospective payment systems, the linkage between patient classification and payment provides an additional incentive for hospital executives to incorporate aggregate statistics from the medical records department in the plans for future operations. Case-based prospective payment systems are valuable in underscoring an explicit association between patient diagnosis and eventual reimbursement.[6-8]

**Figure 9–3** Strategic Management of Medical Records and Billing

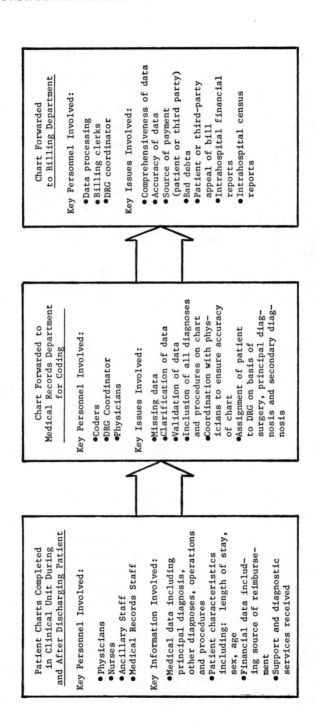

Patient Charts Completed
in Clinical Unit During
and After Discharging Patient

Key Personnel Involved:

● Physicians
● Nurses
● Ancillary Staff
● Medical Records Staff

Key Information Involved:

● Medical data including
  principal diagnosis,
  other diagnoses, operations
  and procedures
● Patient characteristics
  including: length of stay,
  sex, age
● Financial data includ-
  ing source of reimbursement
● Support and diagnostic
  services received

Chart Forwarded to
Medical Records Department
for Coding

Key Personnel Involved:

● Coders
● DRG Coordinator
● Physicians

Key Issues Involved:

● Missing data
● Clarification of data
● Validation of data
● Inclusion of all diagnoses
  and procedures on chart
● Coordination with phys-
  icians to ensure accuracy
  of chart
● Assignment of patient
  to DRG on basis of
  surgery, principal diagnosis and secondary diagnosis

Chart Forwarded
to Billing Department

Key Personnel Involved:

● Data processing
● Billing clerks
● DRG coordinator

Key Issues Involved:

● Comprehensiveness of data
● Accuracy of data
● Source of payment
  (patient or third party)
● Bad debts
● Patient or third-party
  appeal of bill
● Intrahospital financial
  reports
● Intrahospital census
  reports

## Patient Charts in the Clinical Unit

The strategic management of medical records begins even before the patient record is forwarded to the medical records department. Patient charts are maintained in the clinical unit while a patient is in the hospital and completed there after the patient has been discharged. Patient charts contain, for example, data on clinical procedures performed, dietary needs, and changes in medical status. The key personnel involved at these times are physicians, nurses, ancillary staff, and medical records staff.

Physicians are a critical factor in the strategic management of medical records. Because they are responsible for providing the clinical services, they are also ultimately responsible for documenting the precise chronology of diagnoses and procedures on the medical record. Yet, as most hospital executives and medical records personnel recognize, the pressure of providing medical care—its urgencies and complexities—often results in less than complete records. With the express link between diagnosis and reimbursement under prospective payment, however, hospitals cannot afford to permit lackadaisical attitudes toward record keeping among either medical or nonmedical staff.

Many mechanisms are available to ensure that medical staff members are highly conscious of the importance of effectively discharging their responsibilities in the medical records area. Incentive systems, for example, can increase the medical staff's commitment to completing medical records correctly. Hospitals that desire a higher percentage of medical records to be completed by physicians before the patient is released must develop an incentive system that realistically addresses physician compensation, patient diagnosis and treatment, and institutional solvency, if it is to be effective.

The medical records staff usually discovers that it is responsible for gathering information from nurses, physicians, and the heads of ancillary departments when the medical record is incomplete. Although other key personnel are involved, the strategic management of medical records must incorporate incentives to motivate all these personnel to complete medical records promptly. The financial integrity of the hospital is at stake. Delays in the processing of medical records may result in cash flow problems.

Efforts to motivate personnel must be undertaken with an eye toward the type of information needed for each medical record. Information on clinical processes and patient characteristics is essential. Medical data must incorporate principal diagnoses, other diagnoses, operations, and procedures. The need for information on patient characteristics is secondary to the need for accurate information on medical diagnoses, but it must be remembered that final classification into a DRG is based on the patient's length of stay, sex, or age.

## Coding of Medical Records

Once the patient chart has been forwarded to the medical records department for coding (i.e., assignment to a DRG), it should be immediately checked for accuracy. The key issues involved at this stage of the medical records process are

1. acquiring any missing data
2. clarifying any unusual information that may adversely affect the assignment to a DRG
3. validating data when there is room for interpretation and possible upgrading of a diagnosis
4. ensuring that all diagnoses and procedures are charted
5. coordinating with physicians to confirm the accuracy of diagnosis
6. assigning the patient to a DRG on the basis of surgery, principal diagnosis, and secondary diagnosis

At least three categories of staff are involved with the medical record once it has left the clinical unit: physicians, coders, and the DRG coordinator (or someone in a similar position). Physicians and coders must contribute to the accuracy of the record. Although physicians complete their tasks early, they must be available for the inevitable give and take with the medical records department. The complexities of medical care, the unique characteristics of patients, the varied responses of patients to treatment, and the guidelines that differentiate one class of care from another all affect DRG determination. Therefore, the hospital administrator, the chief of the medical staff, and the medical records department supervisor must work together to establish timely and efficient communication on medical records problems.

Responsibilities for DRG coding may be delegated to a DRG coordinator in order to minimize friction between the medical staff and the medical records department. The establishment of the DRG coordinator position itself is a visible indication of the hospital administration's commitment to accurate record keeping and to maximizing the hospital returns from prospective payment. The DRG coordinator not only manages all clinical and nonclinical department efforts to maximize revenues and minimize costs, but also is an advocate for quality of care. Low-cost services that produce malpractice suits or high-cost services that hurt financial solvency are of little value to the hospital.

The DRG coordinator acts as a liaison among departments, integrating and coordinating work to ensure that medical records are complete, that physicians have accurately documented diagnoses, and that DRG coders have the information that they need. The DRG coordinator must be capable of analyzing information flows or standard procedures in order to identify problems before they occur and must formulate specific action plans and recommendations that can be adopted to resolve problems that do develop.

Finally, the DRG coordinator should participate in the ongoing in-service education efforts of hospitals. Specifically, the coordinator should prepare materials to educate staff about the importance of timely and accurate data, and about methods to improve accuracy in completing medical charts. The DRG coordinator must help remove the mysticism surrounding DRGs by presenting clear, understandable diagrams and illustrations of the DRG system. Hospital personnel must understand what DRGs mean in terms of prospective payment and what DRGs mean for their particular department. Once this framework has been developed, the DRG coordinator can manage specific ramifications for a single department or a single clinical task.

## Quality Control

Medical records departments have always been a primary focus of hospital quality control efforts. There has been substantial experimentation with the format of medical records in efforts to improve quality control. Early efforts included problem-oriented systems, which have evolved into the contemporary format that is based on diagnosis and procedure. The structure adopted for the medical records cannot guarantee quality, however; it can only facilitate quality. In the end, there is no substitute for accuracy on the part of medical and nursing staff, or on the part of ancillary department personnel, who document diagnostic and treatment services.

In terms of quality control in the medical records department, strategic management requires a structure around which quality control checks can be incorporated and a system of rewards for personnel who consistently achieve high quality.

### Structure

A quality control structure must be incorporated into the very process by which medical charts are completed and updated. The integration of clinical units with the medical records department, the two areas in which the quality of medical record keeping is most difficult to maintain, is the most important structure. The transfer of the medical record from one unit to another jeopardizes the timeliness and accuracy of the data. Unless quality control checks are established in both areas—clinical and medical records departments—and between the areas, quality may remain elusive.

When medical records must be revised and corrected, other mistakes may be made. The inefficiency itself will be evident in higher costs within the medical records department (although the increase in costs may be negligible compared with the revenues lost as a result of inaccurate record keeping). There is also the problem of the time value of money. Each time there is a delay in the processing of a medical record, reimbursement is delayed. Even one added day's lag in reimbursement for a hospital can be significant when the lost time value of the revenues is considered.

Quality control in the medical records department is also important because the financial projections and strategic planning of the hospital are based on analyses of patient mix and anticipated revenues. Clearly, if a sufficient number of medical records are inaccurate, forecasts will also be inaccurate. Most hospitals have previously established effective and efficient quality control procedures; however, because prospective payment places hospitals at financial risk, it may be necessary for hospital administrators to reassess the quality control procedures in the medical records department to ensure that no changes are needed.

The structure of quality control procedures in the clinical and medical records departments must be very specific. Operationally, the considerations in Table 9–1 reflect the minimal effort that must be invested in maintaining quality control in the flow of information. These ideas are based on the work of Grimaldi and Micheletti, who suggested that some hospitals may wish to include a third element in the quality control process between clinical units and the medical records department—patient accounts.[9]

---

**Table 9–1** Quality Control Procedures and Purposes

| | |
|---|---|
| Nurses must communicate directly with physicians about incomplete patient data or patient orders. | Increases the number of charts that are completed before they reach medical records; uses the greater influence of nurses (compared to that of medical records staff) to full advantage; obtains information from those who are most familiar with patients. |
| Nurses on the clinical units verify daily census figures. | Provides a cross-check on utilization data used in other departments for planning and decision making. |
| Several times each day, medical records department personnel retrieve charts for discharged patients. | Ensures that medical records can be verified and coded with minimum delay and maximum timeliness in forwarding to billing office. |
| Nurses maintain a check system on the medical charts released to medical records personnel, possibly obtaining signatures for charts released. | Provides a cross-check on the location of the charts; encourages responsible handling of charts within and between units. |

**Table 9–1** continued

| | |
|---|---|
| Nurses verify that all diagnostic and treatment services from ancillary services are documented before releasing charts. | Decreases the number of medical records that must be revised before they leave the medical records department for the billing office; ensures proper billing. |
| Operating room personnel maintain a log for definition of surgical procedures completed. | Provides a foundation for correct DRG classification and billing; acts as a cross-check on medical records from the floor. |
| A random sample (e.g., 10%) of medical records is reviewed by the head operating room nurse and the DRG coordinator to confirm accuracy and to compare surgical procedures listed to those on the operating room log. | Implements quality control through statistical sampling. |
| Medical records department receives list of patients discharged daily. | Provides a cross-check on the medical records received from nursing units for patients discharged. |
| Physicians and nurses complete charts, using diagnoses and procedure codes. | Promotes orientation toward efficient classification of procedures; aids DRG classification process. |
| Medical director and nursing director establish and support the policy that all medical records must be completed within four days after a patient is discharged. Financial penalties may be exacted for habitual abuses at either individual or departmental level. | Ensures timeliness of medical record processing and billing. |
| Medical records personnel and DRG coordinator assign DRG. | Provides accurate classification; removes burden of interpreting clinical accounts from billing office. |
| A random sample (e.g., 10%) of cases is reviewed by the medical records department head and the DRG coordinator for proper DRG classification prior to billing. | Provides final confirmation of billing category. |

These operational ideas must be tempered by the nature of the particular hospital and its clinical and nonclinical staff members. These suggestions for control are only starting points from which further structural improvements can be made in the medical records process.

*Rewards*

Incentive compensation is an appropriate mechanism for expressing hospitals' commitment to quality control in the medical records department and billing office. The problems with incentive programs in the medical records department result from traditional payment and compensation. Furthermore, only a few individuals are involved in the accuracy and timeliness of medical records. These are not insignificant problems, and their resolution will challenge even the best hospital executive.

Hospital executives must consider the effect of *not* creating quality- and productivity-based compensation systems, however. If prospective payment is adopted by all third party insurers, the impact of erroneous medical records will be even greater. No hospital can afford to undercut its revenues in such a setting. Thus, it appears that hospital executives have no choice except to design and implement more sophisticated systems of employee compensation that reward or punish fluctuations in the quality of medical record keeping.

Incentive systems vary according to the existing compensation system and the extent to which quality and productivity are to be reinforced. It will probably be necessary to introduce a new incentive program incrementally in order to minimize the number of adverse effects from the modification. Above all, the hospital must recognize that it is introducing a new philosophy that will be difficult to remove once it has been implemented. Careful analysis must be undertaken before such a program is implemented to ascertain cost-benefit sensitivities; the internal costs of the program must be balanced by the benefits that it provides.

In creating the incentive compensation program, the first step is to determine the existing level of quality. For nursing staff, quality may be indicated by the proportion of records for which the medical records department must seek additional information from physicians, nurses, or ancillary departments. For the medical records staff, it may be indicated by the proportion of records that were not correctly coded or were identified as incomplete or inaccurate in the random sample cross-check. Given this base line, administrators and directors (e.g., of nursing and medical records) can begin to establish new quality or productivity goals. Those who perform at the base line level receive no exemplary reward, those who perform below the base line level may receive no annual raise or only a portion of it, and those who perform beyond the base line level share in the cost savings on a percentage basis or from a previously established bonus pool for reward.

In order for this system to have maximum influence, several other operational considerations must be taken into account in the planning process. First, the hospital must plan extensive in-service education to orient the staff to the possibilities of the system. Second, flexibility must be built into the administration of the system. Some coders, for example, may seek those medical records that are easiest to code or prepare for the billing office. The distribution of easy and difficult records must be equitable, however. Third, the system must have a mechanism for grievances that will circumvent any staff member's attempt to play the system for individual gain rather than departmental and hospital gain. The incentive system must be beneficial at all levels—individual, departmental, and institutional.

An effective compensation system is difficult to develop because it requires considerable effort in record keeping and evaluation. This results in higher costs. The question is whether hospitals can afford *not* to implement sophisticated systems that directly address performance. These incentive systems must make it possible to distinguish sources of poor quality and productivity. Many hands touch the medical record in its course from floor to billing, and the incentive system should not penalize medical records staff for the mistakes of other people.

## STRATEGIC MANAGEMENT OF BILLING

A number of critical factors must be managed in the billing department once a medical record or its abstract has been forwarded for processing (see Figure 9–3). There are at least three key staff areas critical to the effective management of prospective reimbursement or other case-based reimbursement systems: data processing staff, billing clerks, and DRG coordinators. Most hospitals have adopted some form of automated medical records system. The data processors are vital in the coding and entering of data into the automated system. Incentive systems for data processors may be appropriate, but the magnitude of the incentives must be tempered by the routineness of the task and the fact that valuable interpretations have already been made in the data.

The DRG coordinator is again a critical management factor in the billing process. The coordinator's responsibility is to troubleshoot deviant cases, to resolve blockades in the processing of records and bills, and to integrate the medical records and billing processes. The power of the position must be reinforced by the top echelons of the hospital in order for the coordinator to resolve any differences between the director of medical records and the business office manager.

The billing clerks are responsible—or at least must be held responsible—for translating the efforts of clinical staff and medical records department personnel into processed bills. The billing clerks must be precise in translating data from medical records or abstracts to patient bills. Copies of the bills will be submitted to the third party payer, to the patient, and to internal files. Errors of any kind can be very costly to the hospital; for example, failure to submit the bill to the correct third party can affect the cash flow of the hospital. Although one mistake may appear to be insignificant, the accumulation of mistakes can hamper financial planning within hospitals.

The billing department must also be alert to bad debts or late payments. Under some prospective reimbursement systems, hospitals may be encouraged to obtain payment for noncovered services from patients. The billing office must keep the admissions office informed about treatments (i.e., DRGs) for which the hospital is seldom fully reimbursed for its costs or for which the hospital must seek incremental supplements from the patient. This area of co-payment remains to be completely resolved, but it appears that third parties will encourage patients to make up the differences between reimbursement and charges. Unfortunately, the burden of collecting the payment will probably fall on hospitals themselves.

The Medicare program does not currently permit appeals of bills, except for errors in calculation or inappropriate application of the rate-setting method. The prospective payment mechanisms adopted by other third party payers may or may not incorporate opportunities for appeal. Obviously, any appeal will severely constrain the cash flow position of the hospital. Although significant policy issues in this area are beyond its control and management, the billing department can help by aggregating data on appeals filed, the aging of accounts because of appeal, and the DRGs under which appeals consistently occur.

Intrahospital census and financial reports must flow from the billing system. Yet, many hospitals have inadvertently developed medical records and billing systems (usually automated) that do not produce a sufficient number of performance quality reports to be forwarded to clinical and nonclinical department heads. In some cases, hospitals have failed to recognize that medical records and patient billing are the foundation behind a management information system. Hospital executives can seldom make good decisions and plans without basic reference to the trends in census and payment. As prospective payment systems are implemented, however, hospitals that have not kept adequate records on patient census and payment parameters will be merely reacting to their environment, not actively taking charge.

## Uniform Billing

The implementation of DRG-based reimbursement may produce some rather unique changes in the format of billing systems. For example, a uniform bill on which the specific charges are identified may be required. The purposes of the uniform bill are (1) to help the third party payer determine the degree of congruence between reimbursement and charges for future rate adjustments and (2) to provide demographic information on patients that can be compared with the original profiles on which the DRGs are based. Specific billing changes will evolve over time. For the moment, the billing office must avoid becoming so regimented that a shift to a new format would be a problem.

Actually, hospitals have reported some very positive benefits from the change to uniform reporting.[10-12] Uniform billing can lead to substantial reductions in data accumulation and duplicate analysis when several payers are involved with a single patient's bill, for example, so that prorating can progress more smoothly (Exhibit 9–1).

### Incentive Systems for Billing

The billing office staff has less responsibility in interpreting medical data than does the medical records staff and probably should be offered a less sophisticated or at least a less extensive incentive compensation package.

Hospitals should consider incorporating patients within the incentive system. Most hospitals have rather archaic billing systems for patient payments. They have traditionally offered patients flexibility in payment plans; too often, however, hospitals have dysfunctionally overlooked the time value of money. Although bills are eventually paid under the traditional policy, the hospital functions as a financial institution that lends money at below market interest rates.

This problem may be exacerbated in the future, since current trends in hospital reimbursement indicate that a higher level of cost sharing through co-payments and deductibles is inevitable for patients. If hospitals expect to minimize the adverse impact of this development on their operations, they not only must upgrade their billing procedures, but also must create a greater awareness of personal financing among admissions officers.

---

**Exhibit 9–1** Uniform Billing for a Patient Covered by Two Insurers. The primary carrier provides benefits of six days room and board and ancillary charges to $300. The secondary carrier pays only for any additional room and board.

| Charge | Primary Carrier | Secondary Carrier | Patient | Total |
|---|---|---|---|---|
| Room and board | $1,200 | $300 | | $1,500 |
| Laboratory | 300 | | | 300 |
| Operating room | | | $200 | 200 |
| Personal items | | | 150 | 150 |
| | $1,500 | $300 | $350 | $2,150 |

If the DRG rate is $2,000, the primary carrier would pay 75 percent ($1,500 ÷ $2,000). The secondary carrier would pay 15 percent ($300 ÷ $2,000) while the patient would pay 10 percent ($200 ÷ $2,000) plus the $150 in personal items.

Hospitals should develop specific payment plans available to patients. They should offer a limited number of financing mechanisms that guarantee payment for dubious cases, but the payment plans must be sufficiently flexible to ensure that final payment will be obtained. Hospitals should also consider expanding the use of cash discounts. Patients are naturally reluctant to pay a portion of a bill that they believe to be covered by their insurance. Hospitals must alert patients to their co-payment responsibilities, providing bills that clearly specify the limits of coverage and the amount for which the patient is ultimately in charge of paying.

Thus, billing departments must work very closely with the chief financial officer and the administrative staff in identifying cash discount trade-offs. A sufficiently large discount may encourage patients to pay more promptly, improving the hospital's cash flow. The number of delinquent payments that become bad debts may also be reduced by discounts to cash-paying patients and sliding scales that offer incentives for timely payment.

## INTEGRATING THE BILLING OFFICE, MEDICAL RECORDS DEPARTMENT, AND CLINICIANS

Although the DRG coordinator works to integrate the medical records department and the billing office, no individual can accomplish the depth of coordination desired for these departments. The main moderating factor is the medical staff. The importance of including physicians in the planning and implementation of plans for managing prospective payment cannot be overemphasized.

Hospital executives must be very careful to avoid suggesting that physicians alone are the cause of inaccurate or untimely completion of medical records. This is just not true in most cases. Certainly, medical records and bills cannot be processed until physicians have completed their patients' charts, however. Billing department and medical records department supervisors are seldom in a position to accomplish much in the way of forceful encouragement with the individual physician. They must work with the hospital administrator in convincing the medical director (or chief of staff) of the deficiencies of any particular medical staff member. With the gentle (and sometimes not so gentle) persuasion of the medical director (or chief of staff), physicians may complete charts as soon as possible on the release of patients.

Departments heads should concentrate on documenting their problem cases. Such documentation can be a constructive basis for discussion. It may involve determining the frequency with which a physician has been late in completing the medical records or identifying the number of times in which the physician had to be consulted (on a per case basis) for explanations or supplemental additions to the record.

In-service education may be the best way to eliminate bad habits in record keeping and to instill in physicians a sense of urgency in regard to the whole medical records process. If this sensitivity is achieved, the goal of integration is likely to be substantially attained. Physicians may be relatively intolerant of the suggestion that they need in-service training, however. After all, every hour spent in training is an hour of lost potential productivity. The medical director (or chief of staff) must present the rationale that, for a very minimal investment of time (i.e., thirty to forty-five minutes over two sessions), the physicians will become much more productive in their record keeping. It must be remembered, however, that the medical director and the hospital administrator are most capable of making these points.

---

**NOTES**

1. David Burik and John G. Nackel, "Diagnosis-Related Groups: Tools for Management," *Hospital & Health Services Administration Quarterly* 26 (1981): 25–40.

2. Roice D. Luke, "Dimensions in Hospital Case Mix Measurement," *Inquiry* 16 (1979): 38–49.

3. Paul L. Grimaldi and Julie A. Micheletti, *Diagnosis Related Groups: A Practitioner's Guide* (Chicago: Pluribus Press, 1982).

4. Ronald Mills, Robert B. Fetter, Donald C. Riedel, and Richard Averill, "AUTOGRP: An Interactive Computer System for the Analysis of Health Care Data," *Medical Care* 14 (1976): 603–615.

5. Susan Dadakis Horn and Dale N. Schumacher, "An Analysis of Case-Mix Complexity Using Information Theory and Diagnostic Related Grouping," *Medical Care* 17 (1979): 382–389.

6. Martin S. Feldstein, "Hospital Cost Variations and Case Mix Differences," *Medical Care* 3 (1965): 95–103.

7. Judith R. Lave, Lester B. Lave, and L.P. Silverman, "Hospital Cost Estimation Controlling for Case Mix," *Applied Economics* 4 (1972): 165–180.

8. James Greenberg and Roger Kropf, "A Case-Mix Method for Developing Health Planning Criteria for Hospital Services," *Medical Care* 19 (1981): 1083–1094.

9. Grimaldi and Micheletti, *Diagnosis Related Groups: A Practitioner's Guide*.

10. John J. Dalton, "Uniform-Reporting Systems for Billing and Discharge Data," *Topics in Health Care Financing* 6 (1979): 62.

11. Carol A. Hyman, "California Hospitals Find Success with Uniform Billing," *Hospitals* 52 (1978): 165–170.

12. Deirdra Bruton, "Uniform Reporting for Case Mix," *Topics in Health Care Financing* 6 (1979): 79–96.

# Chapter 10

# Tactical Factors: Budgeting

Budgets have been abused more often than used in hospitals. In the past, there have been few pressures to bring costs in line with budgeted expectations, and this omission has stimulated higher costs. Both medical and nonmedical departments have been able to escape penalties as a result of excessive costs because their poor performance has been subsidized through other departments. In some cases, hospital executives have come to expect that certain departments will run deficits under virtually any circumstance. This attitude is dangerous at both the departmental level and the organizational level.

Prospective payment requires an entirely new attitude toward operations—and an abrupt halt to runaway costs.[1] Most hospital executives recognize this, but they may not have a clear vision of the best way to resolve the problem. Budgeting can help hospitals develop a framework for containing costs. Surprisingly, budgeting has seldom been integrated into hospital operations as a meaningful cost control mechanism. At best, budgeting methods have been used as guidelines in planning and control functions. Hospitals have traditionally been reluctant to enforce budgets with incentives and disincentives that motivate department heads and program directors, but they must put budgets into such practical use under prospective payment.

## PURPOSES OF BUDGETS

If hospitals are to bring an immediate halt to excessive costs, they must have better mechanisms for managing these costs. Prospective reimbursement encourages an entirely new view toward cost generation, reporting, and control. Budgets can be very useful in all three areas. Budgets can be the basis on which department heads and program supervisors make decisions about their expenditures, for example. The budget provides a profile of necessary expenditures, showing department heads where they must make trade-offs on resource expenditures if they expect to achieve cost control.

Budgets also serve as an effective reporting mechanism, reducing communications about costs into a manageable framework. In this sense, budgets help managers to communicate their expectations. In addition, budgets should contribute to cost control. The primary purpose of budgets is to help managers forecast expenditures and achieve targeted cost and expenditure levels. Control, therefore, is initiated with the planning process.

## PRODUCT LINE ACCOUNTING

Hospitals must upgrade their accounting information systems. This is not an insignificant challenge. It takes years to perfect an accounting system and more years to make it an effective management tool. In the era of reimbursement based on diagnosis-related groups (DRGs) and prospective payments, however, hospitals will be forced to invest in improved accounting systems. Without good data, it will be impossible to determine where costs are generated, when revenues are not offsetting these costs, if one department is adversely affecting others, or whether several departments are experiencing unduly high costs. Hospital executives must take substantive action, resulting in direct and tangible changes in the information and accounting systems.

Some hospital authorities have suggested that the management of prospective payments is similar to product line accounting.[2] For decades, businesses have charted the progress of products by allowing each product to function as a profit center within the overall accounting records. The result has been a more objective analysis of the life cycle of products. Those products for which the net profit is minimal or the marginal costs have not decreased may be deleted from the product line. This sort of analysis is especially valuable when the number of products is large.

The development of newer, more marketable products motivates business managers to analyze a given line of products and to select only the most lucrative for the firm's product line. Such an approach may be increasingly relevant to hospitals. In the broad sense of product line accounting, hospitals have over 467 products (i.e., services) in the form of DRGs. In order to cope with this extensive list of products, hospitals must conduct rigorous financial examinations of each DRG to ascertain where costs exceed revenues—and by what magnitude. They must then decide which DRGs to retain. Once a decision has been made to retain a DRG, the costs and revenues associated with that DRG must be monitored to ensure that it is not replaceable with an alternate, more profitable DRG.

Budgeting and product line accounting are especially compatible because they require the same basic information:

1. the number of patients who use a service
2. the medical parameters associated with use of the service (e.g., disease severity and length of stay)
3. costs of providing the service
4. revenues generated by the service
5. support required from other programs to provide the service
6. contribution of medical personnel to the service[3]

This information is only part of a more sophisticated management control system needed by hospital executives.

Business managers have become accustomed to operating under conditions of financial risk and make resource investment decisions by using objective information on the best methods for reducing costs and improving profits. With the greater financial risks faced by hospitals under prospective payment, hospital executives must adopt this stance. They cannot afford to maintain the standards of the past. Nowhere will changes be as evident as in budgeting, the hospital's operational manifestation of planning and control. Under prospective payment, the cushions and reserves built into hospital budgets will rapidly disappear; in their place, executives must substitute rigorous analysis, objective decision making, forecasting, and institutional control to prevent deficits. Without careful analysis of all the tangible and intangible factors that affect performance, hospitals will discover that they have become incapable of meeting the most basic challenge.

## MANAGEMENT CONTROL PROCESS

The interrelationship among planning, budgeting, and control is depicted in Figure 10–1, which captures the main elements of the management control process as it pertains to hospital operations.[4] Specifically, the external environment places constraints over the goals that hospitals may pursue. Given these constraints, hospitals must define a mission toward which internal operations are directed. Occasionally, these broad goals are implemented through departmental and program budgets, which provide standards against which performance can be assessed. This is the control process.

Prospective payment is a significant environmental shift toward greater constraints on hospitals. Yet, it is only one of the factors that influence strategic planning within hospitals. Technology, ancillary labor supply, availability of physicians, the incidence of disease in a community, competition from other hospitals, and many other factors are also significant constraints over the internal tactical planning and budgeting process.

The limits of external constraints must be taken into account in the internal strategic orchestration of resources. With the imposition of prospective payments,

**Figure 10–1** General Model of the Management Control Process

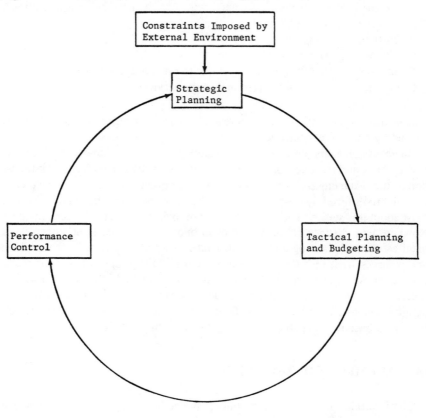

a hospital may discover that it must reduce the scope of its obstetrics department and supporting services, for example, because costs exceed revenue. Therefore, the obstetrics department may delete its parent education programs and its alternative birthing rooms. In addition, because of the impact of the external-internal interface on tactical planning and budgeting, the obstetrics department must prioritize the service elements of its budget. While retaining its main service component, it must either reduce or delete other previously budgeted elements of the obstetrics services. Thus, budgeting functions are the immediate realization of both strategic and tactical planning. The budget becomes the specific operational definition of obstetric services within the hospital.

This example underscores the influence of prospective payment (an external environmental influence) on budgeting (an internal managerial process). The specific budget cuts or additions that result from prospective reimbursement will depend on the hospital, its reimbursement rates, and the extent to which hospital executives are able to develop and manage the connection between external and internal influences.

If prospective payment had necessitated a 30 percent reduction in the operating budget for parent education and alternative birthing rooms in the obstetrics department described earlier, the hospital should assess the impact of this reduction on community interest (i.e., utilization) in obstetrics services after an eight-month trial period. If the number of patients served per month in the obstetrics department has fallen by only 5 percent, costs have been contained. These relationships must be explored further and similar experiments conducted in other service areas where costs are high.

The role of control is to correct deviances in performance. The control process, however, acquires significance from an operationally effective planning and budgeting system in which standards for performance are established in advance of the assessment. Likewise, the importance of budgeting is dependent on control.

Unless these simple, yet productive ideas are included in basic management practice, it may be difficult for hospitals to effect the sort of businesslike results that prospective payment systems require. The history of more lenient approaches to budgeting and control may hamper the implementation of these ideas in some hospitals. If so, hospital executives must work carefully with department heads and program directors through in-service education and personal contact to ensure progress toward better performance.

## PROSPECTIVE PAYMENT AND THE BUDGETING PROCESS

Under prospective payment, the budgeting process takes place in a new context that dramatically affects each of its elements (Figure 10–2). The budgeting process hinges on three critical elements: program plans, estimated demand or activity, and estimated program performance.[5]

### Program Plans

Hospital program plans usually center on direct and indirect patient care provided to both inpatients and outpatients. Prospective payment will affect both inpatient and outpatient care, as well as the plans that hospitals formulate for these endeavors. Outpatient care may increase or change in scope if third party reimbursement provides an incentive to decrease the average length of stay. Physicians may provide more rehabilitative care on an outpatient basis, thereby relieving the hospital of unnecessary patient days, or they may order more preliminary diagnostic tests before a patient is admitted, thereby increasing the return from the

**Figure 10–2** Budgeting Process under Prospective Payment

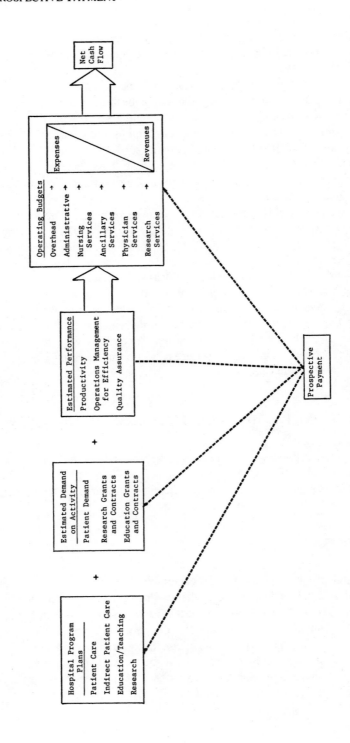

inpatient stay. The extent to which physicians will alter their treatment patterns depends on the incentives and disincentives created by the hospital.

Prospective payment may also alter a hospital's education-related program plans. As third party payers increasingly move their reimbursement systems toward greater cost control, they will impose greater control over education expenses. Hospitals that are affiliated with a university medical school may feel considerable pressure to delete or reduce their level of commitment. DRG-based reimbursement may not cover many (if any) education-associated costs, since in a broad sense, education services do not involve either direct or indirect patient care. Although there are substantial counterarguments, specifically education's importance for the maintenance of quality within hospitals, hospitals will probably be encouraged to reconsider tangential education programs.

Prospective payment will have a similar impact on hospital programs devoted to pure research. Hospitals will be required to demonstrate that these research programs consistently generate revenue from contracts and grants if they expect to maintain such programs under prospective payment. Primary patient care services may no longer be able to produce the surplus funds needed to promote these services. Although the initial phase-in of DRG-based reimbursement appears to be relatively moderate in controlling costs, control may tighten as years go by. Hospital executives must carefully assess research activities for their contribution to overall hospital goals.

Research is expensive and seldom generates more funds than expenses. Unless hospitals pursue research wholeheartedly, however, the funds invested in research programs would perhaps produce more benefits if invested elsewhere. This presents a rather gloomy outlook for research, but it might result in a greater concentration of research resources in medical schools and universities where economies of scale could reduce the costs of research.

## Estimated Demand

The forecasts or estimates of patient demand, research grants and contracts, and education grants and contracts will have a significant influence on the depth and scope of program planning within hospitals. Furthermore, the program plan itself—the precise expenditure of resources on a program—will influence the demand.

If a hospital analyzes its costs for urology-related DRGs and discovers a favorable cash flow, for example, prospective payment can influence both planning and demand. The hospital may undertake a program to expand its urology ward and its staff of urologists simultaneously. Although this decision must be tempered by the incidence of urology-related disease in the community, the supply of urologists, and the competition from other hospitals, it is feasible to expand hospital services in this one clinical service area. Thus, prospective payment has motivated the hospital to revise its plans, which in turn will influence the estimated demand. Prospective payment has also affected the estimated demand directly by establishing a condition (i.e., reimbursement) under which the hospital can benefit by the financial return on its services.

**Estimated Performance**

A hospital program will have a given level of productivity (i.e., output for input), of efficiency, and of quality. Although prospective payment does not generally reward a hospital directly for departmental performance, there is an obvious and necessary relationship between performance and net revenues. Indeed, this is the very essence of prospective payment—to encourage internal hospital efficiency, productivity, and to a lesser extent quality.

**Operating Budgets**

Hospital program plans, estimated demand, and estimated performance are all brought together by the operating budget. Hospital budgets vary extensively from institution to institution, yet most budgets are formed around overhead (i.e., plant and equipment), administrative and general expenses, nursing services, ancillary services (e.g., food services, maintenance, laundry and linen, and laboratory), and to a lesser extent physician services and research services. Operating budgets are based on forecasts of expenses and revenues, as always, but the addition of prospective payment establishes an entirely new setting for budgeting.

## AN OPPORTUNITY FOR ZERO BASE BUDGETING

There is little question that prospective payment presents an excellent opportunity for zero base budgeting (ZBB) in hospitals. In the past, the true applicability of ZBB to health care services has been limited, because most hospitals do not completely review their services every year. They have an accepted component of services that is seldom reevaluated for deletion each year. As a result, ZBB is likely to be more a 20 percent analysis of all services than a 100 percent analysis.

Under a pure form of ZBB, all services are assessed each year for future funding or deletion. Because a hospital must provide certain basic services in nursing, emergency care, laboratory services, radiology services, food service, billing, and related routine services, however, the hospital seldom has the option of deleting these services. Expenditures for these services are not discretionary—they are essential.

Once a hospital has reviewed its optional services—usually centered around patient amenities—it can begin to consider services for deletion. Few hospitals would delete laboratory services, but a large hospital may delete various patient education programs or even a minor involvement in a university teaching program. Hospitals are generally reluctant to cut many optional services, because marketing is often based on these services. Thus, ZBB is a pure concept that is seldom implemented even in the most rigorous situations. Most executives cannot afford the time needed to review all services within a budget. They are forced to differentiate among a relatively small percentage of optional services in making decisions about deleting services.

Prospective payment presents an opportunity for renewed applications of ZBB. Hospital executives must be careful not to overlook ZBB because it did not work in the past or because it appears to be just another management fad. Although it will probably never be a long-run budgeting tool, even under prospective reimbursement, ZBB is a good short-run technique for assessing costs attributable to programs and for determining whether programs should be cut, maintained, or expanded.

## Setting Measurable Budget Objectives

In the ZBB process, the critical point of departure is the setting of measurable budget objectives (Table 10–1). This step reflects the important link between budgeting and planning. A measurable objective for a hospital that must contain costs under prospective reimbursement would be to decrease total nursing department expenses by 10 percent by reducing the number of skilled nursing hours used. As with all good objective setting, a length of time must be specified for the accomplishment of the objective.

The introduction of prospective payment places a premium on effective objective setting. The tendencies of the past to overlook the objective setting process as an unnecessary task must be reversed. Under prospective payment, internal operations must be guided by specific goals and objectives in order to progress toward cost control.

## Categorizing Decision Options

After measurable objectives have been set, the decision options that might be implemented to achieve the objectives must be categorized. In an effort to decrease total nursing department expenses within a hospital, for example, the decision options might include reductions of nursing hours in intensive care, surgery, obstetrics, and extended care. Since nothing is taken for granted in a ZBB analysis, all nursing services must be considered for reduction at first. Because a decision must be made on where a cost control strategy is to be centered, however, hospital executives must develop a rationale (in this example, with the assistance of the director of nursing services) behind the decision options; there must be

**Table 10–1** The Zero Base Budgeting Process

| Step in ZBB Process | Example for Skilled Nursing Care |
|---|---|
| 1. Set measurable budget objectives. | Decrease total nursing department expense by 10 percent by reducing skilled nursing hours used. |
| 2. Categorize decision options. | Decrease nursing hours in intensive care, surgery, obstetrics, extended care. |
| 3. Establish targets of activity. | *Intensive Care*   *Surgery*   *Obstetrics*   *Extended Care*<br>Maintain   → 10%   Maintain   → 20%<br>→ 10%   → 12%   → 5%   → 22%<br>→ 15%   → 15%   → 20%   → 23% |
| 4. Evaluate decision options. | *Intensive Care*   *Surgery*   *Obstetrics*   *Extended Care*<br>Minimum   Fire 0 RNs   Fire 2 RNs   Fire 0 RNs   Fire 3 RNs<br>Desired   Fire 1 RN   Fire 3 RNs   Fire 4 RNs   Fire 4 RNs |
| 5. Rank decision options. | *Priority:*<br>High Priority ↔ Low Priority<br>1. Decrease intensive care nursing hours—fire 1 RN.<br>2. Decrease extended care nursing hours—fire 4 RNs.<br>3. Decrease obstetrics nursing hours—fire 4 RNs.<br>4. Decrease surgery nursing hours—fire 2 RNs. |
| 6. *Implement decision.* | *Decrease nursing hours in  intensive care—save $23,000*<br>*surgery—save $92,000*<br>*obstetrics—save $80,000*<br>*extended care—save $38,000* |

Source: Adapted with permission from Joseph F. Goetz and Howard L. Smith, "Zero Base Budgeting for Nursing Services: An Opportunity for Cost Containment?" Nursing Forum 19 (1980):122–137.

legitimate reasons/criteria for including the respective nursing areas as decision options.

## Establishing Targets of Activity

With the decision options specified, the next step in the ZBB process is to establish targets of activity. For example, after analyzing previous budgeted performance and actual performance, as well as the profitability of various DRGs, the chief financial officer and the nursing director may decide that the nursing hours in surgery should be decreased either 10, 12, or 15 percent. With corollary decreases in other service areas, this'reduction of nursing hours in surgery will allow the hospital to reach its objective of decreasing total nursing department expenses.

Several targets of activity should be proposed for each option. Although this is technically not required, identifying more than one or two target levels helps hospital executives to think about alternatives and to envision a larger program of cost control. This is especially important in the first years of operation under prospective payment. A policy should be established for continuing cost reductions at the budget formulation stage.

## Evaluating Decision Options

Once the targets of activity have been set, the hospital administrator must evaluate the decision options. A likely method to reduce skilled nursing hours and, thus, to decrease nursing costs is to terminate one or more full-time equivalent nursing positions, or portions thereof. Given the targets of decreased activity in extended care, for example, the minimum number of nursing positions that might be terminated is three full-time equivalents, with a desired reduction of four. If reductions are less preferred in intensive care nursing, the *minimum* reduction would be no full-time positions—a decrease in skilled nursing hours could be attained by higher cuts in the other targeted areas. Yet, the *desired* reduction in intensive care nursing is one full-time position. The nursing department must realize that cost control can be achieved only if deliberate cuts in all areas are targeted.

## Ranking Decision Options

After evaluating the decision options, hospital executives must rank them in order of priority. In the nursing hours example, the highest priority would be given to intensive care nursing hours; only one nursing position would be terminated. Then, four nursing positions would be terminated in extended care, four in obstetrics, and two in surgery. This system of prioritization enables executives to differentiate between necessary and desired reductions in the allocation of resources. It also establishes a convenient ordering system should resources become more abundant or should further reductions in nursing hours be required.

## Implementing Decisions

The last stage in the ZBB decision process is implementation. It can be hoped that the number of full-time positions will be decreased through attrition, reduction in the number of temporary personnel, or less frequent use of registry nurses. It is the implementation of the decision, however, that brings with it specific cost savings.

Obviously, similar cost reductions could be achieved very easily by across-the-board cuts of 10 percent in all departments, including nursing services. The advantage of such an approach is that it requires little time and effort (i.e., resource expenditure) from hospital administrators. Furthermore, it is an equitable approach because every department is decreased by an equal percentage. Hospitals that opt for this method will discover that it is very convenient in the short run, but problematic over the long run, however. A comprehensive reduction in all services by 10 percent does not provide a solid foundation for improving operations. It is based on many weak assumptions, the most significant of which is the assumption that every department has slack that must be reduced. Critical departments may be adversely affected, while the truly costly departments merely lose some of their surplus and amenities.

## Overview of ZBB

Many salient features of ZBB have made it a celebrated method for achieving budget control. It presents a wholistic approach to the determination of services provided and services deleted. Such an approach is helpful to hospitals that must respond to DRGs and prospective payment, because these hospitals must begin to formulate a core of strategic services that define the hospital and convey a working identity to the public. In addition, ZBB improves planning and control; budgets are tied to goals and all budget requests (and hence goals) are reviewed before funding is allocated.

The reality presented by prospective payment is that, unless expenses are controlled, deficits will drive the hospital toward financial insolvency. It is evident in Figure 10–3 that not all services can be funded under the proposed budget of this hospital. All hospitals provide only services that support their basic mission. In Figure 10–3, the mission is to provide high-quality inpatient services in obstetrics, general surgery, intensive care, and emergency care. As part of this basic mission, it provides operating facilities and patient rooms (private and semiprivate). Generally, hospitals will discover that they need to specialize in a few services; they will

**Figure 10–3** Zero Base Budgeting and Program Decisions

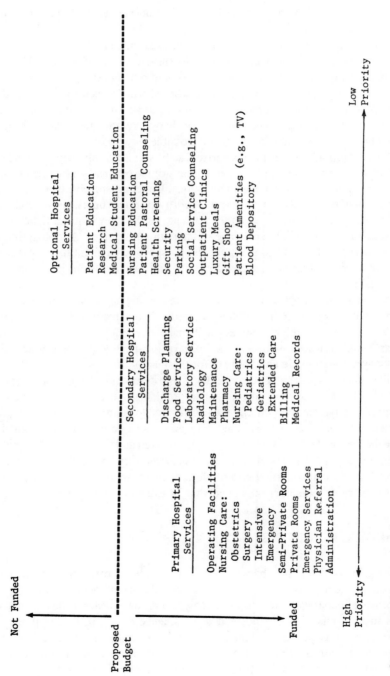

*Source:* Adapted with permission from Joseph F. Goetz and Howard L. Smith. "The Applicability of Zero Base Budgeting in the Long Term Care and Health Services Administration Context,"
*Long Term Care and Health Services Administration Quarterly* 3 (1979):139–148.

probably be unable to perform well (i.e., produce fewer costs than revenues) across all 467 DRGs.

Despite these trends toward specialization, it is unlikely that hospitals will be forced to delete many services in order to survive in the short run. Thus, the secondary services shown in Figure 10–3 should remain relatively untouched by prospective payment. Realistically, if a hospital were forced to delete all these services (perhaps replacing them with contractual substitutes), it is questionable that the primary services could be provided. In other words, there are limits to the retrenchment of hospital services that is possible.

The most propitious area in which to revise the service component of hospitals is the optional service area. Unfortunately, many of the optional services in hospitals are oriented directly toward patient amenities. Under prospective payment, many hospitals will be forced to curtail these supportive services unless the revenues that they produce are at least equal to the expenditures that they require. Patients may be asked to fund a higher percentage of the optional services. Although this will violate many traditional hospital policies, prospective payment has introduced a new environment that necessitates foresight and innovation in the provision of acute and primary care.

The precise services that will be deleted are contingent on the circumstances of the particular hospital. Patient education, research, and medical student education are likely areas in which hospitals will make changes (Figure 10–3). In fact, research and education will bear the brunt of prospective payment unless third party payers incorporate an allotment for these activities.

Like other management ideas, ZBB is most successful when it is applied properly. Because of the constraints and problems that accompany DRGs and prospective payment, particularly the urgent need to control costs and to improve efficiency through service deletion, ZBB appears to be ideal for the short run. Once the cost-ineffective services have been deleted and there is less sensitivity in the entire budget, ZBB will be less effective. At the very least, ZBB helps instill in hospital staff members a better attitude toward planning and control. Hospital executives must remember, however, that ZBB is not a panacea.

## CASE MIX BUDGETING

The primary distinction between budgeting under retrospective payment and budgeting under prospective payment is that the latter incorporates case mix patterns. It encourages executives to analyze alternate scenarios based on varia-tions in case mix. Since a hospital can influence case mix by the process of admissions, it is possible to make one or more of these scenarios a reality, provided that the administration can manage the medical staff and direct the admission of patients whose disease falls within high-priority DRGs.

Admittedly, the administration may have little direct control over the case mix, but by working with the medical director (or chief of staff) and judiciously controlling medical staff privileges, it is possible for the administration to exert considerable indirect control over case mix. Hospital executives may work to help the medical staff internalize the contribution it can make to cost control. Realistically, this is very difficult to achieve without the full cooperation of the medical director in educating the medical staff and revoking staff privileges for excessive costs. Control may be increased by prospective payment systems designed to pay hospitals only and to have hospitals then reimburse physicians, but the strength of physician lobbies will probably militate against implementation of such systems.

Clearly, hospital executives are confronted by a disturbing dilemma. They need to control case mix, because it directly determines all ensuing aspects of budgeting. Simultaneously, they lack the means for effectively achieving that control.

### Centralization vs. Decentralization

The key element of effective budgeting is centralized control. Over the years, however, centralized control has acquired a reputation as inappropriate for most contemporary, large-scale organizations that produce a diverse mix of complex goods and services. The hospital has been used as a classic example of a complex organization that should adopt a decentralized decision-making approach. Large-scale bureaucratization is often inimical to good performance.

The problem with centralization is its tendency to be nonresponsive to the numerous changes at the operations level. If a hospital is administered in an overly centralized manner, patient needs are probably being neglected to some degree because decisions for program changes are delayed. Changes take time, and the hospital personnel most aware of the need to initiate change are powerless to act. If the director of medical technologists in the laboratory observes that outpatients must now wait up to one-half hour to undergo basic procedures (e.g., drawing of blood samples), he or she may convey this fact to the chief executive officer, who may or may not respond to the situation. The chief executive officer is also responsible for other departments, and the operating statistics will not reveal the fine distinction that the laboratory director witnesses. As long as action (e.g., hiring new medical technicians or extending hours of operation on week nights and weekends) can be taken only by top administrators, the hospital reacts less quickly to its dynamic environment.

Hospital executives must approach control cautiously within their organizations. While prospective payment has a highly significant influence on internal operations, executives must recognize that they cannot respond optimally to prospective payment by overcentralizing control in their offices. After all, the hospital's response to prospective payment will be implemented by all (line) personnel. Therefore, excessive centralization will only jeopardize the implementation of departmental budgets (Figure 10–4).[6]

## Central Operations Analysis

Budget determination begins with central operations analysis of six key case mix–related parameters:

1. revenue
2. costs

**Figure 10–4** Budget Determination

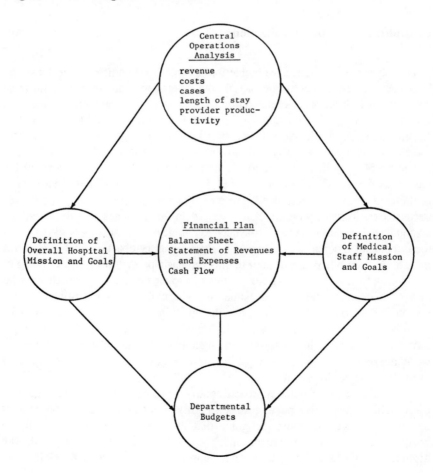

3. cases
4. days
5. length of stay
6. provider productivity

Revenue, costs, patient days, and provider productivity can be considered traditional determinants of the budgeting process. Departmental budgets have always been formulated around a balance between revenues and costs (direct and indirect). Obviously, revenues are associated with the type of patients served (i.e., cases) and their length of stay. Yet, hospital budgets have been concerned more or less with aggregate measures of performance rather than with the fine distinctions that are necessary in case mix budgeting.

Cases, or patient mix, and patient length of stay provide an entirely new dimension for budget determination. The formation and use of the budget are much more complex under DRG-based reimbursement, since the parameters that underlie the budget have been expanded. Department heads and financial staff may be reluctant to give up their past methods of budget management, however, if the hospital executive has not specifically oriented staff to the new budgeting requirements. Essentially, prospective payment requires expanded analysis of *priority* patient mix cases (i.e., those that contribute to excessive costs or abundant revenues for a hospital).

The main goal of central operations under DRG-based reimbursement is to integrate the new factors with traditional determinants in the budgeting process. In the laundry and linen department, the traditional budgeting process may be affected very little. In the nursing department, however, nursing directors will be expected to control costs in those cases in which costs exceed revenues. The two dimensions—cost and case—have made management more complex and challenging.

Eventually, control of budgets should be decentralized. The central staff—the chief executive officer (or representatives), chief financial officer, and medical director—must formulate a plan to prepare hospital staff for decentralized budgeting. Until the hospital staff becomes familiar with the changes wrought by DRGs, it is probably best to continue traditional methods of budgeting with revisions to take DRGs into account. As the staff learns more about the budgets and their new complexion under DRGs, it will be possible to use a more decentralized, bottom-up approach.

The central operations analysis must be incorporated within the definition of overall hospital missions and goals, the financial plan, and the definition of medical staff goals. The DRGs themselves will not serve as the hospital's missions and goals. The board of executives must define a specific mission and realistic hierarchy of goals based on the hospital's resources and the community's needs, although the reimbursement limitations of prospective payment guide the evolution of the mission and goals. Of the financial planning ingredients (i.e., the balance sheet, and the statements of revenues and expenses, and the cash flow), the statements of revenues and expenses are most likely to be altered by DRGs. Physicians are not likely to alter their practice patterns significantly (in terms of either quality or cost), even with the radical shift to prospective payment. It may be possible to influence medical staff missions and goals more extensively in areas with an oversupply of physicians, however. Departmental budgets must be based on changes in cases, length of stay, and provider productivity; the guiding rationale is a rigorous assessment of contribution to net revenues.

Hospitals must move rapidly beyond the conceptual to the specific (Table 10–2). In particular, they must analyze certain data and information in forming their budgets. The greater the precision with which the data and information are collected and analyzed, the greater the accuracy of departmental budgets. Finally, although there is some consistency in responsibility, the degree of responsibility for managing the budgeting process shifts among key executives.[7]

Analysis of DRG data makes it possible for executives to set broad operating goals for the hospital, as well as specific objectives for each provider. The hospital is able not only to establish a budget that guides its activities, but also to establish a mechanism for addressing the variations attributable to its medical staff. Both of these forecasts are essential to the budgeting process. Case mix budgeting,

---

**Table 10–2** Case Mix Budgeting

| Data and Information | Budgeting Issue | Executive Using Information |
|---|---|---|
| Group DRGs by<br>    Revenue (total)<br>    Cases (#)<br>    Days (total patient)<br>    Payer | Which DRGs have the highest priority in terms of service volume and revenue generated? | Administrator<br>Chief financial officer<br>DRG coordinator |
| Group DRGs by<br>    Length of stay<br>    Revenue per case<br>    Revenue per day by payer<br>    Revenue/cost per physician | Which DRGs have the highest priority in terms of medical care delivery and revenue/cost per provider? | Administrator<br>Chief financial officer<br>DRG coordinator<br>Medical director |
| Compare DRGs by specialty<br>    Length of stay<br>    Cost per case (DRG) by<br>        physician<br>    Revenue per case (DRG)<br>        by physician | Which DRGs will produce revenues that exceed costs? Which providers produce revenues that exceed costs? | Administrator<br>Chief financial officer<br>DRG coordinator<br>Medical director<br>Medical staff |

**Table 10–3** Budgeting by DRG

| DRG Number | Average Length of Stay (Days) | Number of Cases This Quarter | Rate | Total Revenue | Cost of Direct Patient Care | Indirect Costs | Surplus/ (Deficit) |
|---|---|---|---|---|---|---|---|
| ×1 | 3.21 | 13 | $ 784.16 | $10,194.08 | $ 9,764.33 | $ 429.75 | $ 0.00 |
| ×2 | 4.33 | 21 | $ 981.98 | $20,621.58 | $16,924.34 | $3,597.24 | $ 100.00 |
| ×3 | 4.12 | 7 | $ 672.47 | $ 4,707.29 | $ 4,011.72 | $ 545.57 | $ 150.00 |
| ×4 | 7.81 | 33 | $1,504.17 | $49,637.61 | $41,711.13 | $6,926.48 | $1,000.00 |
| ×5 | 5.61 | 15 | $ 987.63 | $14,814.45 | $ 8,217.54 | $6,596.91 | $ 9.00 |
| ×6 | 4.37 | 3 | $ 841.35 | $ 2,524.05 | $ 2,000.17 | $ 823.88 | $ (300.00) |
| ×7 | 2.11 | 40 | $ 453.11 | $18,124.40 | $16,733.17 | $1,391.23 | $ 0.00 |
| ×8 | 1.89 | 43 | $ 389.12 | $16,732.16 | $12,897.24 | $1,734.92 | $2,100.00 |
| ×9 | 3.47 | 19 | $ 819.23 | $15,565.37 | $13,464.26 | $2,101.11 | $ 0.00 |

therefore, sets a precedent for overall hospital budgeting and for "product mix" budgeting.

The data collected for case mix budgeting establish a comparative basis for analyzing the specific DRGs and directing attention to problem cases (Table 10–3). They provide a profile on performance, a base line from which problem resolution can begin. They also identify both surplus and deficit so that department heads can begin to scrutinize the internal operations of their departments for critical variables that have jeopardized performance. This is the basic element of budgeting—to forecast performance and to make operational changes that allow the hospital to achieve the budgeted level of performance.

---

**NOTES**

1. "The Abrupt Halt to Unlimited Costs," *Trustee* 36 (1983):28, 30.

2. Marilyn Mannisto, "Managing Case-Mix Reimbursement," *Trustee* 36 (1983):30, 31.

3. Marilyn Mannisto, "Managers Wanted: Case Mix Reimbursement Demands Managers, Not Facilitators," *Hospitals* 57 (1983):91–93.

4. Robert N. Anthony and John Dearden, *Management Control Systems: Text and Cases* (Homewood, Ill.: R.D. Irwin, 1976).

5. Robert A. Vraciu, "Programming, Budgeting and Control in Health Care Organizations: The State of the Art," *Health Services Research* 14 (1979):126–149.

6. For a related treatment, see Susan A. Larracey, "Hospital Planning for Cost-Effectiveness," *Management Accounting* July (1982):44–48.

7. For a related treatment, see David Towne, "Case Mix Planning," *Topics in Health Care Financing* 10 (1983):1–8.

# Chapter 11

# Tactical Factors: The Medical Staff

The era of open-ended funding for health care has now come to a close. During that era, roughly 1946 to 1980, hospital executives focused on setting high charge structures and maximizing patient care volumes. The professional values of physicians to maximize treatment were consistent with the financial goals of hospitals and hospital trustees.

With the growing awareness that the old, retrospective methods of financing hospital care have contributed to the dramatic increase in health care costs, prospective payment systems were developed in an effort to slow the rate of cost increases by changing financial incentives. The effect of this change in financial incentives on cost containment and quality of care will depend largely on the delicate balance of clinical and financial factors on the medical care process.[1]

The medical staff and its leadership will be important elements in the hospital's implementation of an effective tactical plan to respond to the new prospective payment system. Physicians exert a considerable amount of influence over total hospital costs, because they directly control admissions, mode of treatment, inputs and procedures, and length of stay. The advent of prospective reimbursement based on diagnosis-related groups (DRGs) will necessitate an attitudinal change on the part of physicians. Before the implementation of prospective reimbursement, the work of physicians increased the hospital's gross revenues and total reimbursement; now, however, the work of physicians will "consume money."[2]

The new system is directed toward containing hospital costs, not physician charges, which may place hospitals and physicians in an adversarial relationship. The current structure of the DRG payment system contains no incentives for physicians to be cost-efficient. To the contrary, a physician's income will increase with the use of additional ancillary services, tests, and treatments, as well as longer lengths of stay.[3] A physician will derive short-term benefits by maintaining the traditional treatment patterns.

The long-term effect of physicians' continued inefficient treatment patterns will be to jeopardize the hospital's financial solvency. The very survival of the hospital will depend on the physicians' willingness to work within the cost constraints of DRG-based reimbursement. Most analysts believe that physicians must eventually come under a prospective payment system if the plan is ever to achieve its goal of efficient use of health care resources. Until physicians are governed by the same financial incentives that govern hospitals, however, they will find it difficult to change their way of practicing medicine in the hospital setting.

Hospital executives have been urging Congress to bring physicians under a DRG-based prospective payment system as quickly as possible, and Congress has directed the secretary of the Department of Health and Human Services (HHS) to deliver a report in 1985 on the feasibility of such a system.[4] Until a decision has been made to include physicians in the prospective payment system, the hospital's ability to respond to the system depends on the ability of its administrators to gain the cooperation and assistance of the medical staff. Hospitals that have this support in the early implementation stages will survive and prosper, while those without it may be unable to maintain financial stability.

## IMPACT OF PROSPECTIVE REIMBURSEMENT

Under cost-based reimbursement, physicians were largely autonomous; they were isolated from the economic impact of their decisions on their institution. The hospital was held financially accountable for physicians' actions, although it had limited influence over the manner in which resources were combined and utilized to treat various patients. Physician practice patterns that resulted in higher costs were not economic threats to the hospital's financial viability, however.[5]

DRG-based reimbursement creates an interdependent relationship between the hospital's administration and medical staff. Both administrators and physicians have an inherent interest in maintaining the financial viability of the organization. Administrators view this as a direct responsibility, and physicians perceive it as a prerequisite to having a desirable hospital for patient care. As hospital boards look more closely at the resource consumption of individual physicians, it is likely that physicians will become more aware of their own use of hospital resources.

The physician assignment of the principal diagnosis is *the* critical ingredient in prospective reimbursement.[6] Proper and timely completion of medical records is imperative. The physicians and medical records department must coordinate their efforts to ensure the necessary speed and accuracy in completing the patient's chart. Determining the principal diagnosis will require both the clinical skills of the physician and the clerical abilities of the medical records department. Thus, patient care has become both a clinical and an economic exercise in management. Hospitals are being forced to compare their practice patterns with regional and national averages. Medical practice patterns will undoubtedly become more standardized over time.

Under the new prospective payment system, hospitals generate revenue on the basis of discharges rather than on the basis of accumulated charges. It is financially expedient to minimize, rather than to maximize, length of stay and use of ancillary services. Therefore, hospital executives and boards must closely monitor physician practice patterns. Yet at the same time, hospitals must seek physician input to and acceptance of the new system. According to O'Gara, board members, administrators, and medical directors can strengthen physician acceptance of the new imperatives by "supporting the concepts that power is derived from consistency with organizational goals, reinforcing those goals at every opportunity, and rewarding behavior that helps achieve the goals."[7]

## PHYSICIAN CONCERNS AND PROBLEMS

The implementation of prospective payment systems effects fundamental changes in hospital reimbursement and professional relationships within hospitals. Predictably, physicians are concerned about the impact of these changes on the physician role. Physician opinions concerning the new prospective payment system vary widely.[8] At one end of the opinion range are physicians who think that prospective payment systems are a hospital problem, not a physician problem. These are primarily well-established physicians who have large practices and seem unconcerned that DRG-based reimbursement may be extended to them in the future. At the other end are physicians who accept prospective payment systems as a challenge and problem to share with hospital executives. The great number of physicians who attend seminars and teleconferences on DRGs suggests that the latter group may well represent the majority of physicians.

Both physicians and hospital administrators should expect more and more third party payers to adopt prospective payment systems. Blue Cross and other private health insurers will probably follow the lead of the Medicare system in order to avoid cost-shifting strategies. Moreover, if and when physician reimbursement is included in the prospective payment system, Blue Shield is likely to adopt such a system. Similarly, large employers, labor unions, and consumer groups will also begin to seek cost-efficient hospital services. The impact of the new system on hospital financial viability and demand for physician services is uncertain, although it is not expected to be positive. It has been estimated that as many as 1,000 hospitals will be forced to close under the new regulations.[9]

In order to adapt to the prospective system, hospitals will usurp much of the power and control currently held by physicians. The concern that prospective reimbursement will reduce physician autonomy to the ultimate disadvantage of the patient is legitimate.[10] Professional autonomy has allowed physicians to meet the unique needs of each patient, and hospital management should understand and appreciate the importance of this discretion to the professional aspirations of physicians.

Physicians are dedicated to providing the best possible patient care; in their view, cost considerations are usually subordinate to patient needs. Yet, as cost containment becomes essential to hospital financial viability, hospital executives will necessarily become more critical of physician resource utilization. Physicians are concerned that their loss of autonomy and control will cause several quality of care problems. Some expect pressure to admit marginal patients in order to bring down the average cost[11] or to create more complicated diagnoses that qualify for larger reimbursement payments.[12]

Along with the loss of power and independence, physicians also expect the PPS to have an impact on their incomes. As mentioned previously, in 1984 the secretary of Health and Human Services conducted a survey of physician services for inpatients. In 1985, Congress will receive a report on the 1984 survey with possible recommendations for including physicians in the DRG system. Physicians may then be included in the prospective payment system as early as 1986.

Physicians have also expressed concern about the possibility of in-fighting among specialists as a result of shrinking capital investment funds and the need to provide less expensive, cost-efficient health care. Because hospitals will be able to identify the major diagnostic categories or physician specialties that are most profitable, physician groups may be pitted against each other in an attempt to preserve their particular specialty in hospitals.

Hospitals will need to compare individual physicians, single out those responsible for excessive costs, and urge them to change their practice pattern. Yet the data on which administrative judgments will be made have been called into question.[13] Hospitals can buy computer software to do a better job of cost accounting based on real costs and to show how the cost of resources is distributed among physicians. For the first few years of the new payment system, computer information may not include enough details on which the administrator and physician can act. The available software cannot substitute for an information base that profiles the normal use of ancillary care for a particular DRG in the physician's hospital and in other hospitals, yet such norms do not yet exist. Part of the problem in obtaining such information is hospital size.[14] In most of the nation's hospitals, the number of physicians admitting patients in a particular DRG and the number of patients in that DRG are too small to generate valid peer group comparisons for the physicians.

The potential for conflict between physicians and hospital administrators or board members is also a matter of concern. The incentives under the fee-for-service medical payment system, which rewards physicians for doing more, are clearly in conflict with those of the hospital under the prospective payment system. Predictably, some physicians have reacted with anger and fear to the new hospital cost-monitoring mode necessitated by prospective payment.[15] At the same time, administrators are warning physicians that hospitals will go bankrupt without their cooperation. They are refusing to purchase new equipment, eliminating certain expensive procedures, reviewing physician privileges to perform certain other treatments, and revoking the staff privileges of overusers.[16] The net result of these pressures is that the average length of hospital stay has dropped since the summer of 1983.[17]

Yet physicians are very concerned that the new system and the associated pressure to reduce patient length of stay may leave them more vulnerable to malpractice suits. New Jersey has had a prospective reimbursement system since 1979, and conflicts surface constantly. Physicians are liable for early discharge complications. Physicians may want to use a new drug, but hospitals may discourage its use because of cost. Physicians accused of overuse claim that they are protecting themselves against malpractice accusations or treating more complex cases. There is no question that prospective reimbursement increases anxiety levels among physicians.

The future does not promise relief from such physician anxieties. Ten years ago, the physician was the undisputed head of the hospital team, but the growing need for capital and the increasing complexity of medical practice are forcing physicians to share power. Fuchs predicted that competition between hospitals and physicians will increase as the two groups compete for the shrinking health care dollar.[18] Both prospective payment systems and increased incentives for ambulatory care will intensify the struggle for control of health care. According to Fuchs, physicians and hospitals will have to work together to ensure mutual survival.[19] While he believed that they will be able to work out effective compromises, he also forecasted that patients would be the major victims of any failure to compromise.

## STRATEGIES FOR FACILITATING PHYSICIAN COOPERATION

Under a prospective payment system, greater physician involvement in the hospital management team will be necessary in order to bridge the gap between the medical and the financial responsibilities of the hospital. DRGs establish a visible and direct linkage between the practice of individual physicians and the financial stability of the hospital.[20]

### Educational Efforts

One way to obtain physician input and support of the management changes necessitated by the new system is to design an extensive in-house series of educational sessions specifically for physicians. Areas addressed should include

- DRG case mix methodology
- the relationship of DRGs to hospital payment
- potential problems and their proposed solutions
- the effect of prospective payment incentives on the major clinical groups
- physicians' impact on hospital costs, resource use, and revenues
- the importance of timely and accurate documentation

One example is the need for hospitals to provide care in the least costly manner (e.g., the new system may force hospitals to reevaluate criteria for admission to intensive care units). At George Washington University Medical Center, an Acute Physiology and Chronic Health Evaluation (APACHE) preadmission scoring system is currently being developed to measure severity of illness within each DRG and enable providers to evaluate admission criteria.[21]

While educating physicians about the new system is the most effective way to ensure harmonious relationships between the medical and administrative staffs, physicians must also participate in the educational process. At one hospital, a medical staff committee consisting of an internist, a surgeon, and a utilization review expert worked with the hospital's business manager and administrator to develop a computer program that would identify DRG problem areas.[22] One nonphysician, the DRG coordinator, also served on the committee, but he was someone who had already established excellent working relationships with the medical staff. The committee then scheduled noontime lectures about DRGs for the entire medical staff. As a result, there was no animosity or hostility toward the new payment system.

### Physician Participation and Integration

Since physicians are not generally integrated into a hospital's administrative hierarchy, executives must make a concerted effort to ensure physician participation through medical staff organization and leadership.[23] Physicians' acceptance of their new administrative responsibilities hinges on their willingness to identify with the hospital's goals and values. Physician loyalty has traditionally been vested in professional values rather than organizational values. The hospital should not attempt to alter the essential professional values of physicians, but should encourage physicians to adopt organizational values and responsibilities, such as monitoring reimbursement levels and treatment patterns, justifying capital improvements and new technology, determining cost-efficient staffing patterns, and planning for long-term hospital viability. The hospital must realize that physician concerns for quality of care will not diminish. As part of the administrative process, physicians will also be able to maintain and monitor the quality of care.

Medical staff committees and medical staff representation on hospital committees are vehicles for physician participation in the development of operational strategy and the implementation of prospective reimbursement. The medical staff should be represented on the DRG committee to develop the policies to be followed under the new system and to monitor hospital costs. Physician peer review committees can be used to keep physicians informed of particular cost problems and to find ways to solve these problems.

## Data Analysis and Feedback

DRG-based reimbursement provides a natural communication link between hospital executives and physicians in discussing the financial implications of alternate practice patterns.[24] In New Jersey hospitals, discussions between administrators and physicians of DRG cost reports have had positive results. After an initial educational process, most physicians have been cooperative.[25]

Management should provide ongoing feedback on the operations of the DRG system and the hospital's performance relative to that of its competitors. If the hospital is performing poorly, it may be necessary to take additional steps, such as

- a monthly peer review to keep physicians informed about the cost of their treatment protocols compared with those of other physicians
- denial or suspension of admitting privileges
- limits on the number or types of tests certain physicians may order without prior authorization

Before using any of these methods, hospital executives should weigh the costs and benefits of such actions. In general, it is not useful to report a single overly costly case. Hospital executives are not physicians and may not be able to evaluate the legitimacy of additional resources consumed. They do have the responsibility to identify trends toward excessive treatment costs, however, and to inform the medical staff of significant variations from standards.[26]

DRGs facilitate the collection of data useful in demonstrating variations between treatment profiles and patient outcomes. Ideally, this promotes a positive environment in which patients, physicians, and administrators can discuss alternate treatments. Management reports that give information relative to physician treatment profiles for various DRGs also allow administrators and the medical staff to review the economics of their patient care plan (Table 11–1). Such a report showed the medical director at Overlook Hospital in Summit, New Jersey, that the costs associated with one DRG were consistently above standard costs because unnecessarily expensive cardiac pacemakers were being used. Once this was brought to the cardiologists' attention, most were willing to use a less expensive

**Table 11–1** Physician Summary Report for DRG 282, July-December, 1981: Shared Medical Services Memorial Hospital

4/28/82
H-2   DRG   Final No. 282

| Attending Physician Number | Number of Cases | Days Stay | Total Charges ($) | Average Room Charge ($) | Average Ancillary Total ($) | Drugs ($) | Medical Supply ($) | Laboratory ($) | X-ray ($) | Operating Room ($) | Anesthesiology ($) | Respiratory Therapy ($) | Other ($) |
|---|---|---|---|---|---|---|---|---|---|---|---|---|---|
| 1 | 4 | 30 | 7475 | 832 | 1036 | 84 | 58 | 144 | 36 | 347 | 93 | | 271 |
| | | 7.5 | 1868 | | 56 | 6 | 11 | 10 | | | | | 23 |
| 2 | 9 | 64 | 15983 | 789 | 986 | 50 | 47 | 139 | 23 | 311 | 106 | | 308 |
| | | 7.1 | 1775 | | 55 | 4 | 9 | 11 | | | | | 25 |
| 3 | 20 | 193 | 56344 | 1111 | 1705 | 212 | 81 | 366 | 74 | 377 | 99 | 14 | 478 |
| | | 9.6 | 2817 | | 127 | 6 | 14 | 29 | 2 | | | | 66 |
| 4 | 1 | 7 | 1492 | 777 | 715 | 16 | 23 | 63 | | 380 | 68 | | 164 |
| | | 7.0 | 1492 | | 41 | 5 | 4 | 5 | | | | | 24 |
| 5 | 17 | 111 | 28271 | 724 | 938 | 43 | 42 | 143 | 20 | 366 | 77 | | 243 |
| | | 6.5 | 1663 | | 52 | 4 | 8 | 10 | | | | | 24 |
| 6 | 22 | 138 | 36298 | 696 | 953 | 44 | 44 | 141 | 7 | 362 | 92 | | 258 |
| | | 6.2 | 1649 | | 50 | 3 | 8 | 11 | | | | | 22 |
| 7 | 4 | 26 | 5966 | 721 | 770 | 39 | 42 | 133 | | 312 | 57 | | 185 |
| | | 6.5 | 1491 | | 46 | 4 | 8 | 9 | | | | | 21 |
| 10 | 3 | 22 | 5456 | 814 | 1004 | 44 | 30 | 102 | 12 | 363 | 155 | | 295 |
| | | 7.3 | 1818 | | 46 | 3 | 6 | 8 | | | | | 22 |
| 13 | 11 | 63 | 16316 | 635 | 847 | 65 | 53 | 115 | 5 | 343 | 77 | | 186 |
| | | 5.7 | 1483 | | 44 | 4 | 8 | 8 | | | | | 19 |
| 14 | 4 | 30 | 7114 | 832 | 936 | 53 | 81 | 136 | 11 | 397 | 65 | 20 | 179 |
| | | 7.5 | 1778 | | 55 | 4 | 9 | 10 | | | | | 25 |
| Staff | 95 | 684 | 180719 | 807 | 1094 | 84 | 54 | 183 | 26 | 358 | 89 | | 292 |
| | | 7.2 | 1902 | | 66 | 4 | 9 | 14 | | | | | 32 |

*Note:* Line one for each physician is the total, while line two is the average.

Source: Reprinted from *DRGs: A Practitioner's Guide* by Paul L. Grimaldi and Julie A. Micheletti with permission of Pluribus Press, Inc., 160 E. Illinois Street, Chicago, IL 60611, copyright 1982.

model.[27] Physicians should keep the intent of the type of reporting in mind. Reports allow individual physicians themselves to investigate any deviations in their treatment profiles and adapt their practice patterns.

Information from DRG cost reports also enables medical directors, executive committees, department heads, and administrators to monitor medical practice patterns. Medical staff committees should gain importance as DRGs begin to affect the hospital's financial status,[28] and DRG data will supply them with

- individual physician practice patterns, including the use of ancillary services, tests, admission patterns, and lengths of stay (Table 11–1)
- comparisons of physician treatment patterns
- identification of deviant patterns as quality-of-care or cost problems

Many administrators are relying on physicians to help them curb overuse. Peer pressure from physicians assigned to monitor and counsel their colleagues has proved effective because physicians prefer not to deviate from their colleagues' norms.[29]

Although DRG data can indicate the cost of delivering care to specific groups of patients, sources of profits and losses, and the average length of stay per DRG, it cannot reveal why profits or losses occur, who or what is responsible for losses, and whether the existing practice patterns are justified.[30] Therefore, decisions cannot be made solely on the basis of DRG data. Other available data, such as quality assurance, risk management, utilization review, and medical record data, must be taken into account. DRG data only raise questions. The answers can be obtained only by thorough investigation and analysis by physicians and other health care professionals.

## Medical Staff Responsibilities

Physicians have three major responsibilities in the implementation of the prospective payment system. First, they must ensure that appropriate clinical information is included in the system. Leaders of the medical staff should meet with the people charged with designing and purchasing the data system and explain the types of quality indicators that will be needed for cost and quality analysis, such as mortality, frequency of questionable treatment modalities, and length of stay in special care units.

Second, the medical staff must ensure that all diagnoses, procedures, and complications are accurately and legibly recorded. All documentation must be completed at discharge to avoid delays in payment. A medical records committee may be created to monitor data accuracy, or a data control coordinator may be given the responsibility for meticulous coding and abstracting. Medical staffs may also consider amending their bylaws to establish more specific and stringent policies on documentation.[31]

Third, the medical staff must conduct a practice patterns review in order to identify colleagues whose overall pattern of care is costly in comparison to that of others. Such a review requires *both* an adequate number of patients *and* several time periods in order to be representative.[32] Moreover, a physician's practice pattern is subject to many influences. Some patients within a given DRG category may be more seriously ill than the typical patient in this category, and a greater utilization of hospital resources may be appropriate; this can often be determined by reference to the patient's medical records. A high mortality rate may indicate a caseload of more severely ill patients. Review of the physicians' and surgeons' index may indicate whether the high costs of care result from overuse of routine procedures or the use of expensive procedures.

Some hospitals will buy a case mix information system from an outside vendor. The hospital then submits data and receives reports. One such system is MED-COST, which is offered by the Commission on Professional and Hospital Activities. Reports such as the Physician Margin Analysis (Table 11–2) enable the medical staff and individual physicians to compare physicians along a number of dimensions.

### Changing Physician Behavior

Many hospitals have started programs to determine the most appropriate methods to use in changing physician behavior in order to maintain or boost hospital

---

**Table 11–2** Physician Margin Analysis

| Physician | Patients | Total Charges | Average Charge | Average Cost | Average Margin | Total Income | Percent Margin |
|-----------|----------|---------------|----------------|--------------|----------------|--------------|----------------|
| 290 | 19 | $295,030 | $15,527 | $10,163 | $5,364 | $101,926 | 34.5 |
| 201 | 7 | $117,928 | $16,846 | $11,682 | $5,164 | $ 36,150 | 30.6 |
| 499 | 8 | $125,323 | $15,665 | $10,538 | $5,126 | $ 41,012 | 32.7 |
| 200 | 10 | $131,233 | $13,123 | $ 8,237 | $4,885 | $ 48,856 | 37.2 |
| 903 | 12 | $ 20,153 | $ 1,679 | $ 1,454 | $ 225 | $ 2,700 | 13.4 |
| 508 | 25 | $ 28,668 | $ 1,146 | $ 926 | $ 220 | $ 5,512 | 19.2 |
| 79 | 7 | $ 12,069 | $ 1,724 | $ 1,659 | $ 64 | $ 451 | 3.7 |
| 498 | 11 | $ 24,440 | $ 2,221 | $ 2,184 | $ 37 | $ 411 | 1.7 |

*Source:* Reprinted from *How Doctors Can Use DRG Data* by T.G. Dehn and K.M. Sandrick with permission from Care Communications, Inc., Chicago, and the Commission on Professional and Hospital Activities, Ann Arbor, Michigan.

profits, but the results of these programs will not be available until later in this decade. Fortunately, experience has provided hospital executives with several guidelines for dealing with their medical staffs.[33] The most important lesson is that physicians cannot be *forced* to change. They may change their behavior, however, if the change increases their status, educates them, has a scientific basis, produces the same quality of care with less effort, and does not significantly reduce their earnings.

Williams suggested five methods that may be more effective when combined than when used separately:[34]

1. Hospital patient record audit committees can persuade physicians to change their behavior by providing them with data on the costs of clinical practices. When physicians are also given a stake in the change, however, they are even more likely to change their behavior.
2. Various strategies can be used to make it administratively difficult for physicians to carry out the unwanted behavior. For example, the hospital may require certain tests to be ordered in writing rather than through checking boxes on a form.
3. Hospitals may establish financial incentives and disincentives, such as letting physicians share in the profits resulting from cost containment efforts or reducing the salary of physicians who generate unreasonably high hospital costs.
4. Administrators can provide feedback to individual physicians on their clinical decisions.
5. Participative management can be used in all phases of DRG implementation. Studies have shown this approach to be most appropriate for highly skilled people in complex tasks characterized by inherent uncertainty. Physicians involved in all aspects of the hospital's decision-making process on cost containment efforts develop a stake in the outcome.

## APPLICATION OF DATA-BASED CHANGE STRATEGY[35]

The correlation between individual physician decisions and hospital cost control has been documented in one earlier study in which the researchers observed that administrators control very little of the cost variance through management systems improvement; physician norms on admission, length of stay, and course of treatment vary enormously, even for similar cases; and it might be possible to influence physician behavior in hospitals through face-to-face, collaborative strategies.[36] Two main frameworks were used in this study. One was a simple formula for understanding hospital costs developed by Fuchs:[37]

Expenditures = Admissions × Average length of stay × Cost per patient day

Clearly, physicians control the first two variables in the equation. Moreover, these decisions are often made idiosyncratically, since there are no dependable national norms for many common hospital procedures. The third variable in the equation can be considered a function of the hospital's organizational structure. It involves three major groups: patient care group (physicians, nurses, and others who perform hands-on care); support services group (technicians and others who provide required services); and administrative group. The actions of all three groups are most infuenced by physician decisions. This functional view of the hospital's organizational structure provides the second conceptual framework.

Physicians often have a frame of reference that lies outside the hospitals in which they practice. Most are volunteer staff who are free to seek staff privileges at other hospitals. As a result, administrators are justifiably concerned about being responsive and positive in their dealings with physicians.

In order to facilitate physician participation in the management of DRGs, hospital executives must use strategies that are seen by physicians themselves as legitimate, necessary, and useful. Such strategies cannot be based on exhortation; rather, they must be grounded in data provided by physicians and other staff members *themselves* about their daily cost-related behavior. Furthermore, the data should include judgments about the impact of various activities on the quality of patient care, and they should be made available to all hospital staff. This approach requires widespread staff participation in formulating, answering, and discussing questions related to costs and quality of care. Such data-based change strategies have been widely practiced in industry and public school systems for many years.[38]

There are twelve primary components of a data-based, participative change strategy involving physicians:

1. Form a team combining the expertise of physicians, social scientists, change strategist, and researcher.
2. Select a hospital whose administration and medical staff are willing to cooperate in trying new methods.
3. Organize a hospital steering committee of diverse membership, including physicians.
4. Plan the data collection and feedback procedures with the steering committee.
5. Agree in advance that all data will be made available to those who supplied it and that results of the survey will be widely publicized within the hospital.
6. Persuade a variety of hospital staff groups to formulate cost-related issues for inclusion in a hospitalwide survey.
7. Visit individual physicians in their offices to solicit issues to be surveyed.

8. Write, test, and refine survey questions.
9. Distribute the survey to *all* hospital personnel, including the medical staff and trustees.
10. Organize computer printout data into easily interpreted formats for discussion.
11. Feed back the data to the steering committee, selected medical staff, and administrators for interpretation, preliminary problem solving, and the next step.
12. Plan systematic feedback and problem solving with all interested groups within the hospital.

The major purpose of this approach is not to gather objective data on hospital practices that tend to increase or decrease costs, but rather to establish staff members' *collective perceptions* of issues that must be resolved in developing cost containment plans.

In one hospital, a priority item identified by physicians, nurses, and administrators was that new patient admissions were slowed by late patient discharges. Unnecessary hospitalizations, unwarranted lengths of stay, illegible physician orders, and other communication breakdowns between physicians and nurses were also identified as general problems that adversely affected costs or quality. Based on these data, the medical staff and administration developed specific proposals for resolving the problems identified. Until these research results were available, there had been no great receptivity among medical staff for the needed changes. This survey process, however, had created a commitment to change and set expectations for change.

---

## NOTES

1. James Studnicki, "Regulation by DRG: Policy or Perversion?" *Hospital and Health Services Administration* 28 (January-February 1983): 102–110.

2. Emily Friedman, "Getting to Know Us: Hospitals May Finally Learn about True Cost and Pricing," *Hospitals* 57 (March 16, 1983): 74.

3. Lynn Kahn, "Meeting of the Minds: Hospital/Physician Diplomacy Crucial under Prospective System," *Hospitals* 57 (March 16, 1983): 84–86.

4. U.S. Congress, Public Law 98–21 Washington, D.C.: U.S. Government Printing Office, April 1983.

5. Robert A. Connor, "A Management Strategy for Prospective Case-Based Reimbursement," *Health Care Management Review* 6 (Fall 1981): 57–63.

6. David Wirtschafter, "The Impact of DRG's on Medical Management," *Alabama Journal of Medical Sciences* 21 (January 1984): 86–95.

7. Nellie O'Gara, "Trustees Shift Focus: Prospective Payment Encourages a Board's Integrative Skills," *Hospitals* 57 (March 16, 1983): 88–90.

8. David W. Young and Richard B. Saltman, "Medical Practice, Case Mix, and Cost Containment," *Journal of the American Medical Association* 247 (February 12, 1982): 126–133.

9. Gerald E. Bisbee and Henry J. Bachofer, "Usefulness of Case-Mix Systems as a Tool in Hospital Management Must Be Determined," *Federation of American Hospitals Review* 13 (May-June 1980): 37.

10. Young and Saltman, "Medical Practice, Case Mix, and Cost Containment."

11. Marlene Z. Bloom, "Prospective Payment To Alter Relations between MDs and Hospitals," *The Hospital Medical Staff* 12 (June 1983): 22.

12. Karen Hunt, "What the New Congress Will Do to Doctors," *Medical Economics* 60 (1983): 37–51.

13. Michael Nathanson, "Computers Crank out DRG Cost Data, but How Valid Is Information? " *Modern Healthcare* 13 (September 1983): 160–164.

14. Ibid.

15. Jennifer Bingham Hull, "Hospitals and Doctors Clash over Efforts by Administrators To Cut Medicare Costs," *Wall Street Journal* (January 19, 1984): 33, 55.

16. Ibid.

17. Ibid.

18. Victor Fuchs, discussed in Linda Punch, "Payment Changes Pit M.D.'s vs. Hospitals," *Modern Healthcare* 13 (May 1983): 38–40.

19. Ibid.

20. Young and Saltman, "Medical Practice, Case Mix, and Cost Containment."

21. Cynthia Wallace, "Fixed Payment Rates Force Hospitals to Reassess ICU's," *Modern Healthcare* 13 (May 1983): 46–48.

22. Carol Keenan, "Physicians' Opinions on PPS Vary Widely," *Hospitals* 57 (December 16, 1983): 24.

23. U.S. Department of Health and Human Services, *Report to Congress: Hospital Prospective Payment for Medicare* (Washington, D.C.: U.S. Government Printing Office, December 1982): 17.

24. Richard F. Averill and Michael J. Kallison, "Prospective Payment by DRG," *Healthcare Financial Management* 3 (February 1983): 12–22.

25. F. Kevin Tylus, "A Look at DRG Reimbursement in New Jersey," *Hospital Topics* 59 (July/ August 1981): 25–28.

26. Paul L. Grimaldi and Julie A. Micheletti, *Diagnosis-Related Groups: A Practitioner's Guide* (Chicago: Pluribus Press, 1982): 152.

27. Charlotte Rosenberg, "Payment by Diagnosis: How the Great Experiment Is Going," *Medical Economics* 59 (May 10, 1982): 245–256.

28. Thomas G. Dehn and Karen M. Sandrick, *What Doctors Should Know about DRGs* (Chicago: Care Communications, 1983): 10.

29. Hull, "Hospitals and Doctors Clash."

30. Dehn and Sandrick, *What Doctors Should Know about DRGs*, 5–6.

31. Ibid., 9–10.

32. Ibid.

33. Nathanson, "Computers Crank Out DRG Cost Data," 164.

34. Sankey Williams, discussed in Nathanson, "Computers Crank Out DRG Cost Data."

35. This section is based on an experiment reported in Marvin R. Weisbord, James U. Stoelwinder, and Charles H.P. Pava, "Involving Physicians in Hospital Cost Containment: Developing an Action

Research Strategy," *Journal of Health and Human Resources Administration* 6 (Summer 1983): 23–45.

36. Marvin R. Weisbord and James U. Stoelwinder, "Linking Physicians, Hospital Management, Cost Containment, and Better Medical Care," *Health Care Management Review* 4 (Spring 1979): 7–13.

37. Victor R. Fuchs, *Who Shall Live?* (New York: Basic Books, 1974).

38. David A. Nadler, "The Use of Feedback for Organizational Change: Promises and Pitfalls," *Group and Organizational Studies* 1 (June 1976): 177–186.

# Chapter 12

# Tactical Factors: The Nursing Staff

The health care industry today is a system in transition. New prospective payment guidelines have been developed to control hospital costs, and the efficiency of a hospital's nursing operations will be a key determinant of the success or failure of its cost containment efforts. The nursing service is the largest department within hospitals and generally consumes the largest portion of the hospital budget.[1] Consequently, the nursing service comes under particular scrutiny in cost containment policies. As case mix reimbursement is implemented, those who manage nursing service departments will be called on to operate more efficiently while providing quality patient care.

Successful decentralization of the hospital's cost-monitoring system from the financial office to the various departments depends on top management's dissemination of information reports tailored to the individual department's needs.[2] The hospital must conduct seminars to ensure that its nursing staff understands the computer reports. Even more important, however, is the nursing administrator's aggressive effort to acquire the appropriate management skills and take an active role in the transition. As a result of its continuous contact with the patient community, nursing is the leading edge of a quality assurance program. If nursing administrators can demonstrate that quality nursing services can be provided with a lower budget through better management, they will become key allies for hospital executives in their campaign to contain costs and improve quality.

The impact of prospective reimbursement on nursing services is unclear at this time. Much depends on how nursing administrators respond to its challenges. Either nurses will become the most important members of the patient care team, with increased responsibilities for helping to boost their hospital's revenues, or they will become victims of budget-chopping administrators who seek to cut hospital costs by replacing nurses with lower paid technicians and aides.[3] This latter approach could well diminish the quality of patient care and ultimately be more costly.

Nurses, as well as consumers, fear that hospitals will subvert the intent of prospective reimbursement by reducing the size of their staff indiscriminately, classifying as many patients as possible in high-priced diagnosis-related groups (DRGs), increasing admissions of patients who can be treated at low cost, and discharging patients early and readmitting them. The American Nurses' Association warned that

> if the DRGs do not accurately reflect degrees of nursing care needed in each category, it is possible that hospitals will attempt to cut back on nursing care for some patients. And in an effort to save money, RN staffs may be cut or less-skilled help utilized.[4]

California set the pattern late in 1983 when its legislature established a price-competitive scheme for Medi-Cal based on contracting for services and preferred provider organizations. Hospitals promptly started closing units and reducing the size of their staff. Many Massachusetts hospitals are reacting to a recent all-payer pricing system by placing a freeze on hiring and slashing staff positions. During the summer of 1983, several Florida hospitals laid off registered nurses (RNs); one Fort Lauderdale hospital cut the pay of fifty critical care nurses, most of whom had been lured from out of state with bonuses.[5] Finally, some hospitals have been pressuring their older nurses to resign.

## AREAS OF REFORM

Although many hospitals overreacted to the prospect of prospective reimbursement initially, there are some obvious areas of reform within nursing that could improve *both* efficiency and effectiveness. One study showed that as much as 47 percent of a nurse's working time is spent on nonnursing activity.[6] The employment of nonnursing personnel to perform these duties would save money. In addition, if the nursing job were broken down into patient-related and non-patient-related duties, a more accurate picture of nursing costs could be drawn. Excessive overtime is another problem that is being addressed in many hospitals.

Excessive or inappropriate staffing can also lead to inefficiency and higher costs. Staffing is inappropriate when there are too many or too few RNs on the staff. An inadequate number increases the length of stay since the correct level of care was not given; the result is higher costs. While some hospitals are moving to an all-RN staff, others are reducing the size of the RN staff by attrition and using more licensed practical nurses (LPNs). In some places, in-service education is also being cut.[7]

Nurses' response to the pressures generated by DRGs have taken three forms: legal, legislative, and managerial. In 1983, the nurses' associations in the states of

Massachusetts and Washington sued their respective rate-setting commissions, claiming that the rate-setting limits put a disproportionate burden on nurses. A fundamental issue is the documentation of both nursing service costs and nurses' contribution to revenues.

The American Nurses' Association has urged Congress to mandate a system that takes into account the variations in services provided by nurses and to require that the costs of hospital nursing services be made a separate line item in accounting. Several states have already taken steps in that direction. The most advanced is New Jersey's experimental plan for clocking the nursing time needed for patients in different DRGs in terms of "relative intensity measures." The biggest legislative victory for nurses has been a new Maine law that requires hospitals to calculate nursing costs for patients in different classifications and to report these data annually to the state's rate-setting commission. Both New Jersey and Maine now require hospitals to show the cost of nursing services as a separate item on each patient's bill.

These projects free nursing costs from the lump per diem rate. Their practical significance is that the nursing role in reimbursement will now be clearly documented. These data will permit the nursing service to demonstrate its contribution to the generation of revenues on a particular DRG. If nursing costs remain invisible, nursing personnel will remain an anonymous asset to be sacrificed in any time of retrenchment.

## MEASURING NURSING COSTS AND REVENUES

Traditionally, nursing care costs have been grouped with a number of other costs in an overhead amount and distributed evenly to each patient through routine charges. If the DRG payment rate is broken into units that reflect department services used by a DRG, however, nursing administrators will be better able to compare the standard and actual costs of nursing services per DRG. For example, nursing administrators would add the payment amounts allocated to nursing for the DRGs assigned to patients on their unit for a one-month period in order to obtain standard costs. By comparing this standard to the actual monthly unit expenses, nursing administrators could identify variances and seek the reasons for them.[8]

### Cost Determination

There are at this time no nursing cost data that the Health Care Financing Administration (HCFA) or any other payer can use to establish nursing costs per case. The present Medicare law does not mandate a breakdown of nursing service costs; however, recent developments suggest that such a requirement may be imposed as early as 1988.[9] The HCFA is currently funding several projects that are designed to identify and isolate the costs of nursing services. Even if the federal government decides not to reimburse hospitals for the cost of nursing care, cost accounting for nursing services is necessary for the management of hospitals under DRG-based reimbursement.

The productivity of the nursing service can be determined by comparing the cost of providing nursing care for each DRG served by the hospital.[10] It will be obvious how much was made or lost on hysterectomies as compared with that made or lost on Cesarean sections, for example. By comparing the nursing costs for a given DRG treated by the same physician with similar ancillary services for each patient, the financial effects of nursing care per se will be evident. Specific procedures or treatments can then be examined in terms of cost-effectiveness and patient outcomes.[11] Since several nursing units are likely to provide care for the same DRG, it is also possible to compare the costs incurred and results achieved by different nursing staffs.

There are a number of ways to determine nursing costs.[12-14] Some hospitals calculate their nursing care costs in detail. Others prefer the simpler system of coding daily nursing intensity for each patient and tracking the result by diagnosis.[15] All hospitals accredited by the Joint Commission on the Accreditation of Hospitals (JCAH) already have a nursing acuity system for determining staffing needs; this system can also be used to assess costs by DRG. A daily acuity rating for each patient is recorded for the entire hospital stay and can be converted into the number of nursing hours spent in delivering and documenting direct patient care. The levels of acuity are determined by the patient's classification. The nursing costs include salaries and benefits for all the staff on the unit, plus a factor for indirect costs. Since the Medicare reimbursement rate is based on a group of hospitals in the same geographical area and on costs incurred in a base rate year, profit or loss can be compared with those of previous years and those of other hospitals that are nearby.

## Apportionment of Nursing Costs among Patients

The most appropriate and/or accurate method of apportioning nursing costs among patients on the basis of resources consumed is the topic of much debate in the nursing profession. Currently, several methods are being discussed and researched.

### Per Diem Method

Under the per diem method, total nursing costs are divided by the total number of patient days, producing the nursing cost per patient day. To determine the nursing cost per case, the cost per patient day is multiplied by the average length of stay.

In order to allow for some differentiation, patient days can be divided into three categories: (1) surgical, cardiac, and intensive care; (2) normal newborn nursery; and (3) all other areas.[16] The per diem method can also be adapted to reflect the DRG system if nursing costs per patient day are derived from a specific DRG. The simplicity of this approach is a major advantage; its inability to reflect patient care needs or to specify nursing care by type or amount of resources consumed is a major disadvantage.

## Per Case Method

Nursing costs can also be apportioned on the basis of costs per case by discharge diagnosis. The longer the average length of stay, the greater the consumption of general nursing units of service. A study by Caterinicchio and Davies resulted in an empirically derived, case mix-adjusted, patient-specific length-of-stay statistic that can be used to apportion nursing costs.[17] Therefore, the estimation of nursing units of service based on length of stay reflects the relative amount of nursing inputs and corresponding costs of direct patient care consumed by any patient in any hospital. The investigator's method can be used to apportion direct patient care nursing costs based on the case diagnosis.

## Nursing Diagnosis Method

Nursing diagnoses can be used as measures of nursing care consumed. Unfortunately, the literature on this approach is scant, but studies are currently being conducted by Stanford University and the American Nurses' Association.

Curtin proposed that several nursing classification schemes be integrated to determine the amount of nursing time needed to provide care to patients.[18] According to her model, there are twenty-three major nursing care categories to correlate with the twenty-three major diagnostic categories. The nursing care categories are then subdivided into 356 general nursing strategies to correlate with the (then) 356 DRGs.

With this approach, all patients must be classified daily according to both nursing functions necessary for each level of care and the tasks required to carry out the function. The time needed for each task is then totaled to determine the minutes necessary for each nursing function. The daily classifications are averaged over the patient's length of stay; indirect care measures are assigned on a percentage basis, according to the patient's average classification. The final average number of minutes assigned to each DRG/nursing care strategy is determined by averaging the number of minutes of direct and indirect care required for the patient's average nursing classification. After the amount of nursing time needed per DRG/nursing care strategy has been determined, a dollar figure based on the hospital's average salaries for nursing personnel per unit is calculated.

*Intensity Measures*

Horn, Sharkey, and Bertram have developed a method of adjusting costs based on the severity of the patient's illness.[19] Since their severity index was developed to quantify all patients, it does not specifically include an adjustment for the complexity or intensity of nursing care required. In an attempt to remedy this problem, Horn and associates are working to develop a nursing intensity index that will correlate with and refine their sixth intensity variable—degree of patient dependency. If this is accomplished, the average cost of nursing care determined under a detailed patient classification system could be weighted according to its percentage of the total costs for the patient's severity level.

*Relative Intensity Measures*

One of the earliest and most visible methods developed to allocate nursing costs is based on relative intensity measures. The intensity of nursing care increases during the early stages of hospitalization, reaches a maximum at some point, and declines as the patient recovers and is prepared for discharge.[20] Thus, the number of minutes consumed, the amount of resources utilized, and the cost of care are directly related. Research findings on this approach are currently being used to establish reimbursement rates for nursing in New Jersey.

As with other allocation techniques, the absolute minutes are not used for apportioning costs.[21] Rather, an arithmetic abstract serves as a proxy for charges in describing nursing resources used. The calculation process involves three phases: (1) identifying the cost of a relative intensity measure, (2) determining the number of relative intensity measures per case, and (3) calculating the average nursing resource use per DRG. In essence, the cost per relative intensity measure is the relationship between the hospital's total actual nursing costs and the number of minutes of nursing time used by the recipient of care.

Relative intensity measures comprise a hospital cost allocation model that provides a patient-specific, aggregate, internal measure of nursing resources consumed. Although it initially came under heavy criticism, this approach has become a major method for allocating nursing costs among patients and for establishing future rates for DRGs.

*Patient Classification Systems*

For the past decade, many hospitals have utilized patient classification systems as a valid measure of the intensity of care required by patients. Since most nursing departments already utilize a patient classification system for determining patient needs and allocating nursing resources, it is logical to utilize such a system in determining costs of nursing services provided to patients in a particular DRG.

In one of the earliest studies on this approach to apportioning the cost of nursing services among patients, Maher and Dolan grouped patients into three groups: self-care patient, moderate care patient, and total care patient.[22] They then proposed that each day a patient was in the hospital be allocated to one of the three classifications and that fixed and variable costs be calculated for each day. The fixed cost is based on the indirect services provided to the patient by the nursing service department (e.g., proportional cost of nursing administration). Fixed costs were computed for each patient by dividing the total indirect cost by the bed capacity of a particular unit. The variable cost is based on the direct services required by a patient (e.g., feeding and treatments). Observational time studies provide data on the number of nursing care hours used per patient per category, and the number of nursing hours per patient day for each level of care can be determined from this information.

Based on these data, each nursing unit is identified as a cost center, the smallest functional unit for which cost control and accountability can be assigned under the existing accounting system.[23] According to Maher and Dolan, this approach provides accurate data on the actual costs of nursing services for patients in acute care hospitals. As such, it also provides an accurate basis for rate setting, third party reimbursement for nursing services, efficient use of human resources, adequate patient care, and equitable billing.

Many hospitals are currently using various other types of patient classification systems to allocate nursing costs. The GRASP system of patient classification may best lend itself to expansion to a DRG-based system for assigning costs because standardized minutes of care have already been assigned for many nursing activities. The Rush-Medicus patient classification system or any other time-based patient classification system can also be adapted to a DRG-based system.[24] Recent research at Stanford indicated that a time-based patient classification system can also be used to determine nursing resource usage.[25] If a hospital already has a patient classification system in place, the assignment of nursing costs by DRG will be an easier task.

The nursing administrator should develop a patient classification system that not only is appropriate for the nursing case mix, but also parallels the medical classification system developed for the DRG system.[26] This is a prerequisite for cost-effective, high-quality nursing. Nursing care costs should be determined according to patient diagnosis (DRG), patient age, intensity of nursing care required, and personnel who provide the nursing care. The patient classification system employed must reflect the intensity of care needed and provided to patients. Furthermore, it must allow the nursing administrator to predict the nursing care costs associated with the kinds of cases treated in the hospital. The patient classification system is the first step in identifying the nursing service as a revenue-generating center. An examination of nursing practice by DRGs makes it possible for a nursing staff to identify its unique and valuable services and to determine whether it generates more revenue than it consumes.

## Revenue Determination

The nursing service must continually demonstrate that, even though it consumes the largest single percentage of the hospital's operating budget, it also produces substantial revenue for the hospital.[27] Without nursing personnel, the hospital cannot provide the necessary care for patients and will suffer a consequent loss in revenue (closed beds). Validating the benefits of the nursing service in relation to the costs of providing that service requires an in-depth evaluation, however, in which costs per unit of service are related to patient care outcomes such as reduced lengths of stay, reduced rates of patient readmissions, and reduced turnover and absenteeism among staff members. Table 12–1 is a simplified mini-income statement that could be used to analyze the general economic impact of nursing services on the hospital.

It is important to note that nursing in general has held down its costs. One recent study showed laboratory costs increased 80 percent while nursing costs increased only 26 percent over the same time period.[28]

**Table 12–1** Nursing Unit Mini-Income Statement Prototype

| | |
|---|---|
| Revenue: | |
| Private | $1,438,248 |
| Medicare | 686,384 |
| Medicaid | 114,072 |
| Total | $2,238,704 |
| | |
| Expense: | |
| Salaries | $1,329,810 |
| Supplies | 95,213 |
| Total | $1,425,023 |
| | |
| "Profit" | $ 813,681 |

*Source:* Adapted from "Legislation and New Regulations" by Roxane B. Spitzer, *Nursing Management* 14 (February 1983): 15, with permission of S-N Publications, Inc., © 1983.

## INCREASING PRODUCTIVITY

In reacting to the potential loss of revenue associated with prospective reimbursement, hospitals have several options: offset the revenue losses through productivity gains, shift revenue losses to other payers, obtain revenue from non-patient care activities, and/or reduce the quality and accessibility of services.[29] The most desirable option is obviously to increase productivity. Such increases in productivity will be necessary for any hospital that wants to gain or retain a competitive advantage. Monitoring of the nursing department productivity, coupled with the development of performance standards and subsequent corrective action for any deviations from the standard, will help to achieve productivity goals.

### Productivity Definition and Measurement

Debate continues on whether the productivity of nursing services should be defined in terms of the patients' condition at discharge (patient outcomes) or in terms of the care processes administered to patients.[30] The nursing process can be largely attributed to nurses, however, and is largely free from the influence of other health care providers. Furthermore, to some extent, productivity can be determined from the nursing process data obtained from patient classification systems and quality assurance instruments widely used today. The JCAH requires both of them. Since they are both in place in all accredited institutions, their use to measure productivity is attractive.

Dennis, Dunn, and Benson have proposed an empirical model for measuring nursing productivity in acute care hospitals: "Nursing productivity is measured as the ratio of nursing output (in terms of nursing services required) to nursing input (the number of nursing hours actually expended) modified by a nursing quality factor."[31]

There is no single formula that provides a comprehensive measure of nursing output. The professional nature of nursing is such that productivity cannot and should not be measured without the continuing involvement of nurses. The measurement and application of productivity should correspond to the general goals of the nursing department and must be made clear to the entire staff.

Measurement should not be an end in itself. Its principal purposes are to determine current productivity and to evaluate staffing policies. It can also be helpful to the nursing administrator in planning for the future. The next step must be an analysis of the highly discretionary aspects of the nursing process so that the measurement tools can be modified to account for these distinctive components of paid professional work.

## The Nursing Management Report[32]

The most useful tool for nursing managers to increase productivity in a prospective pricing environment is the management report. Generally, these are sent to both fiscal officers and directors of nursing services. The basic purpose is to compare the particular hospital to state averages in terms of various financial and other data for each DRG category.

Table 12–2 shows a prototype nursing management report. Column 1 identifies the DRG by number with the English description alongside in column 2. Column 3 indicates the number of cases in each DRG in the hospital. It is important to monitor overall volume by DRG and trends in such volume in order to better respond to changing demand patterns.

Column 4 indicates how each particular DRG ranks within the particular hospital. For example, in Table 12–2, the sixth most admitted patient is in DRG 039. This assists the administration in quickly identifying the predominant patient diagnosis in their particular institution and helps determine resources necessary to efficiently handle these patients.

Column 5 describes where the hospital falls in comparison with all other hospitals in the state for each DRG. The data in Table 12–2 indicate that the particular hospital treats a relatively high number of cataract patients (DRG 039) than most other hospitals.

The single most important statistic in this report is in column 6, which indicates the average length of stay for each DRG. The average length of stay for DRG 039 in this hospital (H) is 3.34 days, compared to 3.25 for all hospitals in the state (S). Length of stay is a major area in which registered nurses can have a major impact on the entire reimbursement system. By becoming familiar with each DRG's standard length of stay, a head nurse might remind a physician that a patient is coming close to the standard length of stay. The nurse can also check to see if discharge planning has begun and if the patient is ready to go home.

Column 7 indicates the total nursing costs incurred by all patients within that DRG in that hospital. In our example, the most costly DRG is 243 (back disorders). It is unclear why this DRG is so costly since the length of stay is below the state standard.

Column 8 shows the average nursing cost per case in the hospital and in all state hospitals. Again, the nursing cost per case for DRG 243 is much higher than the state average.

Column 9 indicates the nursing cost percentage for each DRG. This represents the percentage of total nursing cost in total DRG cost; in DRG 039, nursing represents 24.69 percent of total costs. DRG 177 represents the highest nursing percentage (64.8 percent). Column 10 indicates how each DRG rates in this hospital with regard to nursing cost. DRG 243 ranks first, or is the highest costing DRG for nursing.

**Table 12-2** Prototype Nursing Management Report

| DRG | Description | Number of Cases | Hospital Rank | State Rank | Average Length of Stay | Total Nursing Cost (All Pts.) | Average Nursing Cost per Case | Percent Nursing Cost of DRG | Nursing Rank All DRGs |
|---|---|---|---|---|---|---|---|---|---|
| 039 | Lens O.R. procedure | 310 | 6 | 9 | 3.34H<br>3.25S | 37,897 H<br>34,747 S | 122.25H<br>112.09S | 24.69 | 15 |
| 243 | Back disorder Medical | 208 | 21 | 21 | 8.50H<br>8.75S | 76,641 H<br>65,099 S | 368.47H<br>312.98S | 49.09 | 1 |
| 177 | Ulcer complications Age 70+ Medical | 14 | 157 | 145 | 9.43H<br>8.85S | 10,640 H<br>7,686 S | 760.00H<br>549.00S | 64.80 | 104 |
| 202 | Cirrhosis and/or alcoholic hepatitis | 23 | 97 | 114 | 12.13H<br>11.00S | 20,360 H<br>16,652 S | 885.00H<br>605.00S | 63.98 | 50 |

*Source:* Adapted from "DRGs: Imperative Strategies for Nursing Service Administration" by R.M. Toth, *Nursing and Health Care,* 5 (April 1984): 199, with permission of Technomic Publishers, Inc., © 1984.

The report tells a nursing administrator to focus upon DRG 243 to find out why it is the most costly in terms of utilization of nursing resources. Possible areas of investigation include inadequate volume of patients; use of temporary nurses; excessive overtime; excessive nurse turnover with resultant higher costs of orientation, education, and down-time; different and more costly treatment protocols; and the provision of non-nursing functions by nurses. Thus, the report has inherent potential for creative managers who are not afraid to investigate what is happening within their department.

In the case of DRG 243, the hospital had nursing costs per case significantly above the state average while the average diagnostic ancillary cost per case (not shown) was below the state average. Nursing was cross-subsidizing ancillary services. Those hospitals in which nursing is well over the average tend to show ancillary services well under budget. One way this problem can be solved is for the nursing department to bill (i.e., housekeeping) for non-nursing services provided by nurses. Another alternative is for the nursing department to take back more of the traditional nursing services such as respiratory therapy or physical therapy. In most cases, it is less costly to have an RN perform these functions along with a broad range of other functions than it is to hire a specialist.

## Productivity Improvement Strategies

In a recent interview, a group of Healthcare Financial Management Association members responsible for planning and implementing hospital programs for DRG management noted that there will be increased emphasis on the development of productivity standards for evaluating hospital departments.[33] Several reported that efforts to involve employees had generated many cost-saving suggestions and that employers are responding to the challenges of reducing cost. Increased use of department incentives to improve productivity was suggested as an important step toward increased employee participation.

Although productivity measurement currently focuses on department functions, improving productivity on a per case basis will require additional attention to the timeliness and coordination of various department activities. For example, procedures to ensure prompt laboratory testing could help reduce length of stay. There will be an increased demand for management engineers and other productivity specialists. Multihospital systems will have an advantage in that they can attract personnel with these skills, but such personnel may also be available to free-standing institutions through shared services arrangements.[34]

### Nurse Staffing

The area that holds the greatest potential for cost savings may be nurse staffing. More hospitals are beginning to schedule and control nurse staffing according to patient acuity levels. Analysis of nursing functions may reveal that less expensive labor can be substituted for more expensive labor. RN, LPN, and nurses' aide ratios may be adjusted to achieve a more appropriate and cost-effective mix of personnel.

The issue of nurse staffing is quite controversial. In recent years, the trend toward increased use of RNs and reduced use of LPNs has accelerated,[35] leading to higher nursing salary expenses. Consequently, some hospitals are now replacing RNs with lower paid LPNs and technicians to cut salary expenses. According to one study, over 40 percent of nursing time is spent on nonnursing activities; therefore, it makes a great deal of sense to increase the ratio of LPNs to RNs.[36]

The major criticism of replacing RNs with LPNs and aides is that the quality of care will suffer because the less skilled employees cannot provide the same wide range of services that RNs can provide. Some studies indicate that replacing RNs with LPNs can actually result in fewer problems, however. One study of eighty-one nursing staff members in seventeen hospitals indicated that the fewest medical problems occur when the staffing mix includes at least 25 percent LPNs.[37] This is consistent with findings of an earlier study that showed little variation in patient care outcomes over a great variety of staffing mixes.[38]

In contrast, other studies have shown that staffing with more RNs can actually reduce costs because the time needed per patient is decreased.[39,40] One study showed that an RN staff using nursing diagnoses and assigned by the case method (rather than by tasks) provided better care at lower cost than did a staff that included LPNs and aides.[41] It is also possible that the length of stay is decreased, when RNs provide care, thus generating additional cost savings.

Obviously, the issue of nurse staffing is a complicated one for which all the data are not yet available. Even if an optimum staffing level and skill mix were determined, there are other considerations, such as union relations and the availability of RNs.[42]

*Product Lines*

Short-sighted hospitals will try to improve productivity by reducing the size of their staff. The long-run impact of this approach could be lower productivity, however, because morale might be damaged and outstanding personnel might start looking elsewhere for a job with security. The more forward-looking hospitals will determine the services that they provide most efficiently and will specialize in them. As a result, there will probably be fewer "full-service" hospitals in the future.[43]

Just as industry uses cost accounting to determine the actual cost of producing various product lines, each hospital must determine the cost of each service (nursing, laboratory, dietary, and medical records) that is included in the cost of treating each product line (DRG). Initially, hospitals should calculate the actual cost of providing care for their highest volume DRGs, identifying all the resources that these DRGs are consuming. After deciding which units of service are necessary, the hospitals should focus their attention on controlling the cost of the necessary service units.[44]

Eventually, the productivity effort will turn to an analysis of services that could be provided at lower levels of care. There are now so many competitive options available that, if a hospital does not move in that direction, it will see a steady decrease of its traditional patient base.

*Behavior Change*

Some hospitals are taking a decidedly behaviorist tack, rather than a management engineering approach, in their productivity improvement efforts. At Memorial Hospital System, a three-hospital organization in Houston, the emphasis is on new thought processes and the quality of work life.[45] Management brought in a consulting firm to teach positive reinforcement techniques to hospital supervisors. Special educational programs on leadership styles for supervisors, the effect of productivity improvement on profits, expansion, and job security for workers are conducted by top management. In addition, a productivity committee composed of hospital executives develops new projects for long-term productivity improvement. The organization is also beginning to tie pay increases to performance appraisals. While formal productivity measurement has not yet been implemented, the Memorial Hospital System believes that productivity is improving as a result of better attendance and reduced overtime.

There is now some evidence that hospital workers are becoming more concerned with the quality of their work life.[46] They want jobs that will use their minds, allow them to grow, give them a voice in decision making, and offer them choices in benefits, hours, and dress. Redesigning jobs to give employees less rigidly defined jobs and wider areas of responsibility can enhance the quality of work life, but it may require management to relinquish long-established traditions. Management may find it necessary to adapt organizational structures to the needs of workers, rather than requiring workers to adapt to organizational needs.

Increasing management's productivity may be difficult.[47] Most management training programs offered by hospitals are inadequate. Consequently, managers should periodically assess their own performance. Hospitals should reexamine the training needs of their executives and the effectiveness of their training programs.

A fundamental tactic to improve the quality of employees' work life is to give them greater control over their work. The single most important factor in nurses' job satisfaction is their perception of having control over their own practice.[48] There are four change processes that can help nurses maintain and increase control over their work while responding to the need for cost containment:[49]

1. Information about prospective reimbursement and its impact should be provided to nurses.
2. The involvement and participation of nurses in productivity improvement programs should be widespread.
3. The strengths of the existing situation should be used, and the fewest adaptations possible should be made. Administrative acknowledgment and reinforcement of these strengths motivate staff members to make changes and try new ideas.
4. Expectations should be clarified and in-service education provided.

Productivity improvement groups, or quality circles, are an excellent way to involve staff members in increasing productivity.[50] Quality circles are employee groups formed to examine problems with a demonstrable cost factor and to decrease waste, duplication, and unnecessary procedures. While each circle chooses the problems it will work on, several issues are quite appropriate, such as tailoring staffing patterns to the needs of the unit, determining the most cost-effective skill mix, and making nursing care plans more effective. The task is to research the problem and find a way to save money. The administration must implement the proposals for change in order to keep staff involved in the process. One hospital estimated that it realized savings of $200,000 annually through quality circles.[51]

In addition to employee participation, patient participation can be helpful in cost containment. Many hospitals are investigating programs to improve patient education in the area of self-care. By teaching patients or patients' relatives to perform minor nursing chores, staffing can be reduced. Hospitals should explore various incentives for patient participation, such as reduced bills for those patients who perform such chores.

As previously noted, one of the most serious and significant changes that may face a hospital as a result of DRGs is the necessity of employee layoffs. Obviously, layoffs should be avoided wherever possible and should be viewed as a "last resort" when attrition and other means of personnel reduction costs fail. When such layoffs are necessary, both the prospect and the reality can adversely affect employee productivity. Hospital executives or nursing administrators who must manage employee layoffs can minimize such negative outcomes through outplacement programs and other methods of alleviating the human and economic costs.[52]

The increased use of volunteers can also enhance the productivity of permanent employees. Volunteer programs need to be well managed, however, in order to develop and maintain volunteer commitment.[53] The director of any hospital volunteer program should understand the needs that motivate volunteers and take steps to respond to these needs.

According to John Belcher, vice president of the American Productivity Center, "effective productivity improvement strategies are integrated into the management system so they are seen not as a program but as a management process."[54]

Toward that end, top management must be committed to the effort to improve productivity, rewards should be given for improvement in productivity, and clear and explicit responsibility for productivity must be established. In addition, a measurement mechanism must be established to focus attention on productivity. Belcher believes that, "if you attend to all these things, productivity reaches the point where everybody recognizes their responsibility for improving it on a day-to-day basis and it becomes part of the organizational culture."[55]

If hospitals are to measure and reward nurse productivity appropriately in the context of their professional values (discretionary judgment, achievement, commitment, and personal growth), they must base their models on professionally acceptable criteria.[56] Nurses have already established procedure manuals and skill checks, standards of practice, continuing education and shared evaluation models, clinical ladders, and (to a limited degree) models of peer review, all of which are helpful in monitoring productivity.

Professionals need not only sufficient remuneration to support a decent standard of living, but also continuing education, community respect, a workplace that fosters professional standards of practice, and the respect of their co-workers for their professionalism.[57] This combination of factors both rewards and spurs professional productivity. If hospitals adopt "industrial" productivity models that fail to consider the professional values of nurses, industrial models of protection (i.e., labor unions) are likely to be the response.

## MANAGING THE CHANGE PROCESS[58]

Several managerial changes are required in the nursing area as a result of prospective reimbursement.

### Planning

The shift of the nursing department from a cost center (viewed as an ancillary expense) to a revenue center is crucial to the future of the nursing profession. In order to accomplish this, nursing administrators need more control and autonomy over the financial management of their departments. Presently, most nursing administrators must request budget allocations from higher administration, which makes the budget unpredictable and severely limits the planning process. Nursing administrators will need significant political skills if more autonomy is to be gained, however.

Since financial resources will become increasingly scarce and more difficult to obtain, nursing administrators must also develop the skills to forecast departmental needs and develop a budget based on forecasted needs.[59] Until they gain more autonomy, nursing administrators will also need solid negotiation skills to ensure procurement of necessary resources. An ability to present nursing needs in appropriate financial terminology will also be helpful. In addition to developing the necessary skills for planning the nursing budget, nursing administrators should be concerned with planning on a hospitalwide basis.[60] The nursing department's own resource needs require that nursing assume a significant role in the strategic planning process.

## Organizing

Decentralization tends to be greater under prospective reimbursement, but this decentralization does not create more conflicts or coordination problems.[61] Department heads simply exert greater influence on their department's operating rules and procedures. The nursing department's operating rules and procedures are more specific and more strictly enforced. The net impact is to diminish the time demands on the head of the nursing department, help lower level nursing administrators to function as true managers, and involve staff nurses in decisions about their department. Such involvement (once accepted) often leads to higher productivity, improved quality, and increased organizational commitment.

## Staffing

A valid patient classification system is a basic necessity in the control of staffing. Without a patient classification tool, budget and/or staffing cuts will be based on assumptions or imprecise data.[62] The use of a valid classification tool will help to ensure the nursing staff's accountability, implementation of the best staffing patterns, and the most effective delivery of nursing care.

## Directing

All nurses should be familiar with the technical aspects of DRGs, as well as with the behavioral and attitudinal changes that prospective payment requires of nurses. Educational programs must also give nurses the knowledge and skills required to provide quality care efficiently. Furthermore, steps should be taken to develop the leadership and managerial skills of first-line nursing administrators, since they are so crucial to the success of the hospital as a whole. The development of these leaders requires programs in all nurse management functions and roles.

## Controlling

If the hospital does not already have a computer system that integrates management and patient care information, the nursing department should urge the hospital to acquire such a system.[63] With prospective payment comes a growing demand for accurate and complete documentation of services and costs.

The nursing service should also regularly develop, gather, and present department statistics that are current, clearly organized, and readily available to nursing and hospital leaders. Such information should include nurse/patient ratios, occupancy rates by unit, hours of nursing care expended on each unit, budget data, turnover rates, salary data, and productivity data.[64] Without such data, nursing management tends to lose control. Finally, nursing service should take definitive steps to control nurse staff involvement in nonnursing activity.

### Implementing Change

In order to survive under the new system, nursing and other department administrators must respond proactively to the pressures of prospective pricing. This requires an acceptance of the necessity for change, an ability to persuade others to change, and an ability to develop realistic implementation plans.

Exhibit 12–1 is a convenient checklist that can be used to guide the change process. Health care administrators who are successful as organization change agents are likely to be good planners who are sensitive to and capable of managing all phases of the change process.[65] They should be not only skilled in the reinforcement of positive behavior and in the use of power, but also comfortable in dealing with conflict and resistance during the change process. Finally, they should have good group and interpersonal communication skills, including the art of listening.

## STRATEGIES FOR THE NURSING PROFESSION

Nursing must be ready to meet the inevitable challenges of increased competition inherent in the prospective payment system. The profession may develop goals in the legislative, educational, and research areas.

Nursing practice should be clearly defined in the Nurse Practice Act to reflect the realities of current practice.[66] Increased political lobbying is also a necessity in order to develop a sphere of influence and power that can be used to increase consumer choices and support direct payment by third party payers to nurses and other nonphysician health care providers. Innovative methods to communicate directly with the public should also be explored.[67]

The high level of collaboration that is required between nurses and other health care professionals under prospective payment necessitates greater educational preparation on the part of nursing administrators. Nursing administration has become the most significant of nursing specialties in terms of its impact on the profession and its input into future management decisions. The team approach to

**Exhibit 12–1** Checklist for Planned Change

| (Yes) | (No) | |
|---|---|---|
| _____ | _____ | I have identified or awaited the occurrence of a problem creating a felt need for the change. |
| _____ | _____ | I have anticipated conflict as a result of gathering data preceding the change. |
| _____ | _____ | I have anticipated resistance to a change that is selected from among a number of options. |
| _____ | _____ | I have provided information that gives direction to those affected by the change. |
| _____ | _____ | I have anticipated resistance to change from those persons receiving such information. |
| _____ | _____ | I have minimized the use of coercive power and restricted its use to trying to unfreeze old habits. |
| _____ | _____ | I have anticipated conflict when using coercive power. |
| _____ | _____ | I have taken full advantage of reference power to facilitate the change process. |
| _____ | _____ | I have provided open and two-way communication with all persons affected by the change, and plan to maintain this communication during the entire period of the change process. |
| _____ | _____ | I have provided extra resources to persons and departments in need in order to support the change. |
| _____ | _____ | I have provided special incentives to reinforce the desired change and to increase the satisfaction of those who succeed with the change. |
| _____ | _____ | I have obtained top management support for the change; this commitment is clear to all persons affected by the change. |
| _____ | _____ | I am skilled at interpersonal communications and group dynamics. |
| _____ | _____ | I am comfortable dealing with conflict. |
| _____ | _____ | I am willing to listen to sources of resistance to change, and to constructively modify the change based upon feedback provided. |
| _____ | _____ | Appropriate corrective action or contingency planning has been taken for every "no" response on the checklist. |

*Source:* Reprinted from John R. Schermerhorn, "Guidelines for Change in Health Care Organizations," *Health Care Management Review* 6 (Summer, 1981): 15, with permission of Aspen Systems Corp., © 1981.

management requires nursing administrators who understand problems not only from a departmental perspective, but also from an institutional perspective.

In addition to information about prospective payment systems, education for nursing must focus on the vast role that computers and information processors will play in management. Nursing will increasingly be identified as a business, and nurses will need a more managerial perspective on their role.[68] They will need more knowledge about economics, administrative theory, organization behavior, finance, and marketing.

There is also a great need for nursing to market itself and to educate the general public concerning nursing's role.[69] Therefore, the services that nursing offers should be compared to those that the consumer really wants or needs, as determined by a community assessment.

Research has been an area of deficiency in nursing.[70] The transition to diagnosis-related descriptions will make nursing research more case-oriented. In particular, research must be undertaken to document the difference that nursing makes, for example, in reducing length of stay, and the need for correlating case mix and nursing diagnosis. Studies analyzing nursing care cost-benefits are timely and essential.[71] Quality, efficiency, and cost containment must be linked through research.

---

## NOTES

1. Jane Meier Hamilton, "Nursing and DRGs: Proactive Responses to Prospective Reimbursement," *Nursing and Health Care* 5 (March 1984): 157.

2. Franklin A. Shaffer, "Nursing: Gearing Up for DRGs. Part II: Management Strategies," *Nursing and Health Care* 5 (February 1984): 97.

3. "DRGs Make R.N.s More Important—Or Too Costly," *Modern Healthcare* 13 (May 1983): 44

4. "The DRG Revolution Gets Rolling: Hospitals Already Cutting Back," *American Journal of Nursing* 83 (November 1983): 607–621.

5. Ibid.

6. "DRGs Make R.N.s More Important—Or Too Costly."

7. "The DRG Revolution Gets Rolling."

8. Richard T. Fox, "DRGs: A Management Control Tool in Hospitals and Multi-Institutional Systems," *Hospital Progress* 62 (January 1981): 53.

9. Leah L. Curtin, "Cost Accounting for Nursing Services," in *DRGs: The Reorganization of Health*, ed. Leah L. Curtin and Carolina Zorbage (Chicago: S-N Publications, 1984), 201–206.

10. Sallie M. Olsen, "The Challenge of Prospective Pricing: Working Smarter," *The Journal of Nursing Administration* 14 (April 1984): 24.

11. Ibid.

12. Paul Grimaldi and Julie Micheletti, *Diagnostic Related Groups: A Practitioner's Guide* (Chicago: Pluribus Press, 1983), 155–166.

13. Susan Horn, Peter Sharkey, and David Bertram, "Measuring Severity of Illness: Homogeneous Case Mix Groups," *Medical Care* 21 (January 1983): 14–22.

14. Curtin, "Cost Accounting for Nursing Services."

15. Olsen, "The Challenge of Prospective Pricing: Working Smarter," 24.

16. Curtin, "Cost Accounting for Nursing Services," 20.

17. Russell P. Caterinicchio and Robert H. Davies, "Developing a Client-Focused Allocation Statistic of Inpatient Nursing Resource Use," *Social Science and Medicine*. In press.

18. Leah Curtin, "Determining Costs of Services per DRG," *Nursing Management* 4 (April 1983): 17–19.

19. Horn, Sharkey, and Bertram, "Measuring Severity of Illness."

20. Paul L. Grimaldi and Julie A. Micheletti, "RIMS and the Cost of Nursing Care," *Nursing Management* 13 (December 1982): 12–20.

21. Ibid.

22. Ann Butler Maher and Barbara Dolan, "Moving Away from the Per Diem Method: A Rationale," *Nursing Management* 13 (September 1982): 17–21.

23. Ibid.

24. Curtin, "Determining Costs of Service per DRG."

25. Melinda Mitchell, Joyce Miller, Lois Welches, and Duane D. Walker, "Determining Costs of Direct Nursing Care by DRGs," *Nursing Management* 15 (April 1984): 29–30.

26. Shaffer, "Nursing: Gearing Up for DRGs."

27. Roxane B. Spitzer, "Legislation and New Regulations," *Nursing Management* 14 (February 1983): 13–21.

28. National League for Nursing, *Newsmaker* 26 (February 1980): 4.

29. Paul L. Grimaldi, "Public Law 97–248: The Implications of Prospective Payment Schedules," *Nursing Management* 14 (February 1983): 25–27.

30. Shelia A. Wilson Haas, "Sorting Out Nursing Productivity," *Nursing Management* 15 (April 1984): 38.

31. Lyman C. Dennis, M. Dunn, and G. Benson, *An Empirical Model for Measuring Nursing in Acute Care Hospitals* (Chicago: Medicus Systems, 1980), 11–12.

32. This section is based on Rosalinda Toth, "DRGs: Imperative Strategies for Nursing Service Administration," *Nursing and Health Care* 5 (April 1984): 197–203.

33. R.R. Kovener and Michael C. Palmer, "Implementing the Medicare Prospective Pricing System," *Healthcare Financial Management* 37 (September 1983): 74–78.

34. Ibid.

35. "Hiring Too Many R.N.s May Cause Nursing Problems," *Modern Healthcare* 13 (June 1983): 49.

36. Ibid.

37. Ibid.

38. Myron D. Fottler, *Manpower Substitution in the Hospital Industry* (New York: Praeger, 1972).

39. Curtin, "Determining Costs of Services per DRG."

40. E. Halloran, "RN Staffing: More Care—Less Cost," *Nursing Management* 14 (September 1983): 18–20.

41. Edward J. Halloran, "Staffing Assignment: By Task or by Patient," *Nursing Management* 13 (February 1982): 20–26.

42. Olsen, "The Challenge of Prospective Pricing: Working Smarter."

43. Neal Bermas, quoted in Glenn Richards, "Working Smarter: Productivity Takes on New Importance under Prospective Pricing," *Hospitals* 57 (October 1, 1983): 94.

44. Roberta Graham, quoted in Richards, "Working Smarter: Productivity Takes on New Importance under Prospective Pricing."

45. Richards, "Working Smarter: Productivity Takes on New Importance under Prospective Pricing."

46. Addison C. Bennett, *Productivity and the Quality of Work Life in Hospitals* (Chicago: American Hospital Association, 1983).

47. Ibid.

48. Olsen, "The Challenge of Prospective Pricing: Working Smarter."

49. Ibid.

50. Ann Haggard, "Quality Circles," *Nursing Management* 14 (April 1983): 16–20.

51. "Quality Circles Save $200,000: Might Mean Edge in New Payment System," *Modern Healthcare* 13 (March 1983): 64.

52. Myron D. Fottler and Dennis Schuler, "Reducing the Economic and Human Costs of Layoffs," *Business Horizons* 27 (July-August 1984): 9–16.

53. Myron D. Fottler and Carol A. Fottler, "Management of Volunteers in Non-profit Organizations," *Nonprofit World Report* 2 (September-October 1984): 18–21.

54. John Belcher, quoted in Richards, "Working Smarter: Productivity Takes on New Importance under Prospective Pricing," 99.

55. Ibid, 99.

56. Leah Curtin, "Reconciling Pay with Productivity," *Nursing Management* 15 (February 1984): 7–10.

57. Ibid.

58. For a more detailed discussion of some of the material in this section, see Myra Crawford and Myron D. Fottler, "The Impact of Diagnostic Related Groups and Prospective Pricing Systems on Health Care Management: An Overview," *Health Care Management Review* (in press) and John R. Schermerhorn, Jr., "Guidelines for Change in Health Care Organizations," *Health Care Management Review* 6 (Summer 1981): 1–17.

59. Carolyne Davis, "The Federal Role in Changing Health Care Financing," *Nursing Economics* 1 (September-October 1983): 104.

60. Hamilton, "Nursing and DRGs: Proactive Responses to Prospective Reimbursement."

61. Hans Boerma, *The Organizational Impact of DRGs*, vol. 4 of *DRG Evaluation* (Princeton, N.J.: Health Research and Educational Trust of New Jersey, 1983), vii–ix, 50–54.

62. Hamilton, "Nursing and DRGs: Proactive Responses to Prospective Reimbursement," 158.

63. Ibid., 159.

64. Ibid.

65. Schermerhorn, "Guidelines for Change in Health Care Organizations," 16.

66. Donna Richards Sheridan, "The Health Care Industry in the Marketplace: Implications for Nursing," *The Journal of Nursing Administration* 13 (September 1983): 36–40.

67. Ibid.

68. Schaffer, "Nursing: Gearing Up for DRGs."
69. Ibid.
70. Ibid.
71. Sheridan, "The Health Care Industry in the Marketplace," 39.

# Chapter 13

# Tactical Factors: Advice to Department Heads and Supervisors

Many hospital excutives are interested in the impact of diagnosis-related groups (DRGs) and prospective payment on rising health care costs. Cost containment must somehow be translated into specific action by hospitals. These actions usually begin at the top echelons of the hospital with strategic planning and control, but the types of medical decisions made for patient diagnosis and treatment are the fundamental basis for cost containment. Top administrative plans and strategies are secondary to medical decisions in importance for cost control.

Control over medical decisions and strategic administrative interventions may improve financial performance; however, higher or lower hospital costs result from the cumulative effort of all staff members. The role of the ancillary departments (e.g., nursing, food service, housekeeping, social service, physical therapy, security, billing, and medical records) is often overlooked in efforts to contain costs. The cost of a hospital stay per patient day is a result of services provided by these departments—even if more intensive medical care is delivered—this is the base from which high costs begin. Therefore, because hospitals must contain costs if they are to remain financially solvent, ancillary services will be called on to make an equal, if not greater, contribution to cost control than do other areas of hospital operation.

The strategies that are implemented at this level must be oriented to the long run in order to be effective. Many hospital executives will be tempted simply to reduce salary increases, minimize benefit contributions, or decrease staffing to achieve instant cost control. There *may* be some slack in staffing patterns that can be removed through higher employee productivity, but hospital executives should not rely on these quick fixes for cost control among the supporting services departments.

Prospective payment will force hospitals to contain costs at all levels. Hospitals must integrate plans from the top echelons to the operating level if costs are to be systematically controlled, a fact not always acknowledged by the formulators of health policy. Hospital executives are now beginning to realize that they alone are responsible for articulating needed changes in operations. They must orchestrate all resources toward more efficient performance.

This challenge can best be met by effective use of department heads and supervisors. Supervisory staff must be included in the plans for managing prospective payment, as they represent the main source of control over the highest number of employees. They are responsible for daily progression toward cost control. Cost containment may not be as glamorous or exciting at this level as at the policy or strategic management levels in the health field; however, it is a daily reality.

## KEY LEADERSHIP FUNCTIONS

The best way to attain high productivity, efficient service, and quality performance from subordinates has always been to adhere to the key leadership functions. Management authorities have tried for decades to identify the principal functions that characterize the effective leader. One representation of the leadership task involves a meaningful effort in planning, motivating, controlling, and organizing (Figure 13–1). There are often variations on this model, but this set of functions is representative of what is required in the typical hospital setting. Hospital department heads and supervisors must concentrate on these special functions if they want to lead their subordinates, programs, and departments toward more cost-effective performance.

For example, the director of purchasing and materials management must, with subordinates, plan and schedule future purchases to ensure that the optimal economic benefit is obtained from quantities ordered. The director must motivate personnel to cooperate with other hospital departments. The director must organize the tasks of department personnel so that all work is completed and maximum productivity achieved. After all these functions are under way, the director must return to analyze individual and department performance before devising new plans (i.e., strategies and tactics) for improving goal attainment.

When prospective payment is added to the hospital environment and hospitals become even more interested in achieving lower costs, many of the leadership functions are attenuated. Specifically, the planning, controlling, and motivating functions appear to have greater relevance under prospective payment systems. Hospital executives should be aware of this and should ensure that their department heads and program leaders understand it as well. Executives may also consider specific management development programs that improve the ability of their surbordinates to carry out these functions.

**Figure 13–1** Primary Leadership Functions under Prospective Payment

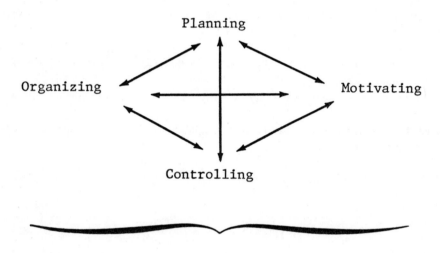

Primary Leadership Functions

Planning

Organizing                    Motivating

Controlling

Functions Attenuated Under
Prospective Payment:

Planning
Controlling
Motivating

## Planning

The one leadership function that probably has the most verbal support, but the least meaningful activity, at supervisory levels is planning. All managers know they should plan, but not all managers make a concerted effort to plan unless the administration is applying pressure for tangible evidence and results. Top management's commitment to and reinforcement of planning is only sporadic in most organizations, and the commitment to planning at the department or program level is unlikely to be any more consistent. These attitudes and reactions must become obsolete under prospective payment.

Prospective payment encourages hospitals to formulate specific goals and objectives with detailed methods for reducing costs and/or improving productivity. Thus, department heads and other leaders not only must allocate time to define the specific plans by which their departments will contain costs over the next twelve months, but also must work with each subordinate to clarify the individual's participation in this larger effort.

For example, the food service manager might formulate a plan that includes maintaining the costs of food and nonfood supplies while improving worker productivity:

1. Maintain expenses for food supplies at the level of the previous twelve-month operating period.
2. Increase worker productivity by 5 percent over the next twelve months.

Then, the leader must work with specific employees in defining these goals as part of their performance criteria:

- Cook: Reduce burned or destroyed/spoiled food supplies by 10 percent over the next twelve months.
- Kitchen Aide: Reduce time spent on cleaning pots by twenty minutes each day, and increase time spent on cleaning trays by twenty minutes each day.

These goals establish a basis for lower costs and higher productivity. Although they do not necessarily control costs in a big way, the cumulative effect of such goals is significant.

Planning has always been a primary leadership function. It will become increasingly important as hospitals are confronted by revenue constraints that drive them to search for cost control.

## Controlling

It makes little sense to expend a greater effort on formulating cost control plans if department leaders fail to follow through by monitoring performance and comparing it to the previously defined standards (i.e., goals and objectives). It is more useful to help cooks and kitchen aides plan for better performance *and* to help them recognize their success or failure in meeting those performance targets.

## Motivating

Department leaders must motivate their subordinates toward improved levels of performance—higher productivity and lower costs. Normally, this is a difficult task. Under prospective payment, it may be even more difficult, since potential economic rewards may become more limited. It is less likely that hospitals will be able to pay the across-the-board wages they have in the past. Pay will be increasingly linked to performance.

## DEPARTMENTAL/SUPERVISORY PLANNING UNDER DRGs

With respect to a hospital's cost control program, planning is a rational process for specifying objectives (Where do we want to go?), determining the present state of affairs (Where are we now?), and selecting the best alternatives for achieving the stated objectives (How are we going to get there?). It is no different for hospital department programs.

Planning the contributions that the ancillary staff can make to cost control involves more than preparing the goals that form a department plan. One of the most important and often most difficult steps is setting specific objectives that include statements of desired future conditions, the time by which they are to be achieved, and the means for measuring them. Although this sounds simple enough, objectives should not be accepted until they have been measured against an established set of criteria.

It is a growing belief in theory and practice that effective goal and objective setting will improve employee productivity and facilitate cost containment. The prevalence of this belief can be seen in hospitals' adoption of goal-setting programs and packages such as management by objectives, organizational development, and performance appraisal. The management and health services literature, however, does not completely support this contention; in fact, it does so only with qualifications. The issue for hospital executives, department heads, and supervisors is whether goal setting positively affects staff productivity and capacity to contain costs.

Analyses of the association between formal goal setting by employees and productivity have shown mixed results. In a study conducted at the Weyerhauser Company in Tacoma, Washington, Latham and Baldes researched the effects of goal setting on the production of logging truck drivers.[1] Two goal-setting treatments were tested, one in which workers were given general directions to "do their best" and another in which workers were given a specific goal of maintaining 94 percent truck net weight. During the first month, the performance of those given the specific goal improved substantially more than the performance of those given the general goal. This increase was maintained over time.

The implications of this study for hospital goal setting and cost containment under prospective payment are clear. Department heads and supervisors must do more than admonish their staff members to "do their best" in holding down costs; they must work with staff members in setting meaningful, measurable targets that provide specific guidance. Without this specificity, staff members are unlikely to change their behavior patterns. Without changed behavior, the goal of cost control is left to chance.

In a similar experiment on goal setting, Latham and Yukl[2] encouraged forty-one typists to set goals for improved performance. The purpose of their study was to determine whether participative goal setting is more effective than assigned goal setting in achieving increased performance. Goal attainment was measured by the percentage of weeks in which the performance of a typist was equal to or better than the goal. There was a significant improvement in the performance of both the group who set their own goals and the group to whom goals were assigned. There was no significant difference between the groups in terms of goal difficulty or frequency of attainment. It was concluded that subordinates' participation in goal setting was not as important as the establishment of a specific rather than a generalized goal.

This finding is very important for hospitals confronting prospective payment. It is a common belief that hospitals need to encourage greater employee participation in efforts to improve productivity and lower costs. Yet, the preceding study suggests that participation alone will not produce the desired results. In and of itself, participation may create a more harmonious working environment, but it does not necessarily contribute to better performance. Department heads and supervisors must go that extra step and establish specific goals.

Ivancevich conducted an experiment to compare participative, assigned, and no training (comparison) goal-setting groups.[3] He used sales personnel to conduct the initial study, and he used 129 skilled technicians and 23 supervisors from seven medium-sized equipment and parts manufacturing organizations to conduct a replication of this study two years later. In neither study was there a significant difference in performance between participative and assigned goal groups. As in other studies, however, there was an indication that specific goals enhanced productivity more than did general goals. Again, the implications for hospitals and their supervisors are clear—cost containment depends on translation of general concerns into specific action.

Kim and Hammer have extended this research by exploring the effect of performance feedback and goal setting on productivity and satisfaction.[4] To evaluate performance, they used four measurements: (1) cost, (2) absenteeism, (3) safety, and (4) service. The results suggested that goal setting accompanied by feedback is superior to goal setting alone in terms of cost and safety performance. The subjective service rating also appeared to be improved by feedback. It was concluded that, although formal goal-setting programs do increase productivity, they are even more effective when accompanied by self-generated knowledge of results plus supervisor-generated knowledge of results and praise. This may be primarily because employees know exactly what is expected from them, how they are doing in relation to those expectations, and what they need to be doing to meet those expectations. It appears that goal setting and feedback decrease ambiguity in the organizational environment.

All of the preceding studies seem to reveal that goal setting increases job performance, but only as long as the goal is attainable.[5] If it is not, goal setting will be dysfunctional and become a source of stress.

These research findings should be applied to the hospital setting under prospective payment. For example, the medical records director who is interested in revenue maximization must help medical records personnel improve the accuracy of DRG assignments. With the cooperation of staff members, the medical records director must establish such a goal and provide periodic feedback on each staff member's performance. Without these basic steps, the goal of accuracy in DRG assignments remains too ambiguous for meaningful action by staff members.

Although the research shows the positive correlation between goal setting and productivity, the employee productivity issue still surfaces in hospitals. Despite the use of goal-setting techniques, productivity and performance still need improvement in many hospitals. Thus, it may be that goal setting is simply an element of the conventional wisdom of organizations, rather than a factor in the improvement of productivity and performance.

## DEPARTMENTAL/SUPERVISORY CONTROL UNDER DRGs

One of the most emotionally loaded supervisory control issues in hospitals today is the issue of performance appraisal.[6,7] It is especially controversial in hospitals because of employee professionalization and the inherent difficulties in evaluating the work of professionals. It is often avoided simply because of the stress that can be created when one person must pass judgment over another. In the final analysis, however, the question is not whether performance appraisal is done; the question is how performance appraisal can be made better to benefit hospital, department, and staff member performance.

The failure of hospital executives to develop objective standards for performance appraisals has resulted in rating systems that utilize broad abstract traits, such as loyalty, attitude, and creativity. These traits have been adopted because they are relatively easy to rate and because they provide a uniform standard that may be used across diverse departments. Furthermore, some performance appraisal systems are designed to identify and penalize relatively insignificant (to the completion of the task) miscues instead of to help hospital employees improve performance through constructive feedback. The foundation for an effective appraisal system is a climate of organizational support, however, not a climate of fear and apprehension.

An increasing number of hospitals are designing performance appraisal systems that alleviate the traditional problems of subjectivity, inconsistency, and employee resistance. This effort will be repaid when hospitals are striving to achieve greater control over departmental and individual performance. One of the first steps in implementing such a system is to convince employees of its merits. Employee awareness of what a performance appraisal system can do *for* them is an absolute necessity if they are to accept it and thereby allow it to work effectively.

## Identification of Critical Job Behaviors

Performance appraisal seldom accurately assesses an employee's *total* performance. It must focus on those selected activities, results, and personal characteristics that enhance productivity on the job. A review of the position description is the natural place to begin when identifying the activities critical to successful job performance. Ideally, every job description is composed of three distinct elements:

1. the actual tasks to be performed, the requirements of the job, and the type of responsibilities. Some position descriptions even suggest how the job activities are to be performed.
2. key result areas. For each performance area, there must be specific, measurable accomplishments that indicate fully satisfactory performance.
3. the personal characteristics essential to successful task completion. This includes the knowledge, skills, and individual traits which enable management to predict the fit between an employee and job.

## Observation and Documentation of Employee Performance

The valid observation and documentation of employee performance is more difficult than most hospital executives predict. For some supervisors, observing employees' performance is a natural function. A charge nurse who continually interacts with the nursing staff, for example, is well prepared to document various aspects of a staff member's performance. The chief executive officer of a hospital chain, in contrast, may have less direct contact with the top administrators of the individual hospitals and, therefore, may be less able to comment on their performance. The main problem is recording notable employee performance when it occurs, rather than waiting until later and relying on memory.

It should not be assumed that the department supervisor is the most appropriate rater. Insisting that supervisors make judgments even if they are not in a position to judge creates pressure to falsify ratings. It may be possible to utilize judgments of peers, clients, subordinates, and, in some cases, of the employees themselves. There are advantages and limitations to each rating source. Perhaps the safest approach, as well as the most valid, is the use of two or more raters who are in a position to observe the employee's performance. This is an expensive and time-consuming approach, however.

Documentation of only the good, or only the bad, aspects of performance will be perceived by the subordinate as threatening and will be demotivating in the long run. It is important to balance the good with the bad whenever possible in order to maintain trust and credibility with the employee. The entire picture must be presented, however, not just the peaks and valleys.

## Preparation for the Appraisal Interview

Good appraisal interviews do not just happen. They are the result of careful preparation by both supervisor and subordinate. From both the supervisor's and the subordinate's perspective, good preparation involves reviewing the employee's file, developing specific objectives for discussion, and determining the desired outcomes of the interview. It might also prove helpful to review the employee's progress with someone from personnel or top management before the actual interview. Frequently, the objectivity of a third party is needed to refocus and remind the parties about the real issues before them.

One of the more difficult tasks in preparing for the interview is designing open-ended questions that encourage the employee to talk freely about his or her results and progress. The art of channeling the conversation without dominating it takes practice. Without adequate preparation and practice, supervisors find themselves engaged in conversation that is unproductive and uncomfortable.

Finally, the supervisor must demonstrate to the subordinate that the performance appraisal process is worthwhile and that the end result is important. If the supervisor is not enthusiastic and confident about the interview, the employee cannot be expected to be enthusiastic and confident.

## Informal Progress Reviews

Unlike the formal appraisal interview, informal progress reviews are excellent opportunities to recognize, discuss, change, and correct deficiencies when they first occur, before they become unalterable. They also allow supervisors to praise performance when the praise will have a more powerful and motivating effect on the subordinate. New employees who are trying to develop good work habits especially need this constant reinforcement from the supervisor.

The frequency of informal reviews may range from as often as once a month to as seldom as twice a year. The employee's need for feedback and the cost of continuing uncorrected performance problems should determine the frequency. Some employees, because of the complexity of their job or their own inadequacies, need to meet frequently with their supervisor. For example, nurses who perform or assist in tasks that must be performed with a minimum of errors (e.g., surgery) need immediate feedback regarding their job performance.

## Formal Review

The formal or annual review session is commonly used to inform the employee of job ratings, merit increases, and promotions. There should be *no* negative surprises at this session; problems should have been discussed as they occurred. Usually, the formal session is designed to establish an overall rating of the employee's performance over a specific period. It is best if the supervisor and the employee can reach a mutual agreement on what the rating should be, but this is not always possible. At any rate, it is the supervisor's duty to accept responsibility for the finalized rating.

Once an overall rating has been discussed, the two parties should focus on the factors that might have influenced the subordinate's past performance. Identifying the strengths as well as the weaknesses that have led to current performance helps to balance the discussion. When discussing specific weaknesses, the supervisor should concentrate on correcting two or three, while minimizing the impact of others.

## Reassessment

The final step in the performance planning and review sequence is a reassessment of each of the elements that comprised the total system. Such a reassessment is made either during or immediately following the formal appraisal session and may include an updating of the job description. Without this final step, the system would be static and could not be adapted to the dynamic health care environment. With this step, however, employees stay attuned to the technological changes, job descriptions remain current, and new objectives are recognized. The key to success, one that makes this system more effective than others, is the involvement of the employee.

## DEPARTMENTAL/SUPERVISORY MOTIVATION UNDER DRGs

After objectives have been set (i.e., planning) and performance appraisal conducted (i.e., control) at the supervisory and department levels, the next step is to translate these efforts into a feasible program of employee motivation. Ancillary department heads and supervisors may have one of the most difficult tasks in the hospital once prospective payment systems have been introduced—the motivation of ancillary department personnel. Neither hospital executives nor middle managers should underestimate the problems that will arise in motivating personnel under DRG-based reimbursement. These problems are essentially those of raising employee productivity (to produce more output for the investment of inputs) and minimizing costs (to enable an overall reduction of costs relative to revenues). There is a dilemma because the new internal environment in hospitals asks employees not only to make do with less, but also to produce more at the same time.

Employee motivation has always been easy in a hospital with more than sufficient resources. Raises at above economic inflation rates have not been atypical and continue to this day. With the implementation of DRG-based prospective reimbursement, however, hospitals will be in an immediate cost bind. Excessive expenditures will have to be controlled. Since labor costs comprise the largest cost area in hospitals, they are very likely to be targeted for budget cuts. Staff will be asked to take less frequent and lower magnitude raises—unless the general cost containment effort of the hospital is successful in reducing costs.

Even if cost control is effective, it is easy to forecast a more restrictive funding environment. Third party payers will determine the rate of increase in DRG payments. Thus, the hospital is at the mercy of these payers to provide an environment in which there is some slack. It remains unclear whether staff salaries and wages will suffer disproportionately compared to other cost areas. The status of unions in a hospital, the history of past wage and salary structures, and the prioritizing of funding cuts will ultimately determine the impact of the new system on employee wages and salaries.

These possible developments are especially detrimental for hospitals that have not developed compensation systems based on performance. If the amount of funding is spread equally over all pesonnel, regardless of performance, then strong performers will be discouraged and ultimately may reduce their level of performance. By contrast, a system tied to performance—whether cost, productivity, quality, or related criterion—prepares employees to accept responsibility for their output. The perfect system will be of little use, however, if there are simply no funds for additional compensation or if the increment is so minuscule that it is a demotivating factor. Although department heads or supervisors may question the probability of this event, the real danger is in not being prepared for the austerity that may accompany prospective payment.

Even though ancillary personnel have never received excessively large increments (compared with those of similar professionals outside hospitals), they have been relatively protected from extremes in fluctuations. Now that department heads and supervisors can no longer count on the motivating power of money, they may discover that it is much more difficult to coax their staff members toward higher levels of performance. On the other hand, the relatively high degree of professionalism among the ancillary staff in most hospitals makes it clear that money alone does not motivate hospital employees. Like other professionals, they are motivated by many other factors, such as the ability to help treat and cure people of disease.

Unless a professional receives fair payment from the hospital, however, the turnover rate will be high. In the past decade and a half, some rural and urban hospitals have had severe problems in nursing turnover; this problem will not be improved by constraints on nursing salaries. When turnover rises, total hospital costs rise because of the added administrative expenses associated with recruiting and retaining personnel. One can only speculate on the ramifications for the quality of care provided under these circumstances.

Supervisors and department heads must be prepared to work with top administrators in designing incentive systems to increase motivation among ancillary workers. As most organization behavior research has indicated, pay on the basis of performance is desirable if compensation systems have been developed to meet the particular needs of a professional group. Thus, a system that is useful for nurses may be inappropriate for food service workers, and vice versa.

## ATTAINING GOAL CONGRUENCY

In view of the funding problems associated with the implementation of prospective payment, hospitals cannot afford to allow any department to optimize its performance at the expense of the entire organization. Hospital departments must attain goal congruency.

The evolving definition of hospital missions and aims is built on a layering of goals (Figure 13–2). Individual goals are the foundation for departmental goals; departmental goals are the foundation for hospital goals. Failure to address the integration of goals is a critical omission. Department heads and supervisors may overlook the need for integration, however, either because they are rewarded for department performance and not for contribution to overall hospital goals, or because hospital executives have neither explained the need for goal congruency nor established integrating mechanisms to achieve this end.

With DRG-based reimbursement, greater attention will be focused on department and work unit performance because of the need to contain costs within budget categories. Unless the emphasis on departmental goals is managed carefully by the top administration, one department may be pitted against another in the race to gain a larger share of the reward pie. As a result, department heads may make decisions that are not in the best interests of the hospital, even though they improve the performance of the individual departments.

Hospital executives can resolve this problem by including contribution to organizational goals among the criteria used to evaluate the performance of the department and the department head. If department heads know that they will be penalized for preventing other departments from performing at their best, they will

**Figure 13–2** Goal Congruency: Evolving Definition of Hospital Missions and Aims

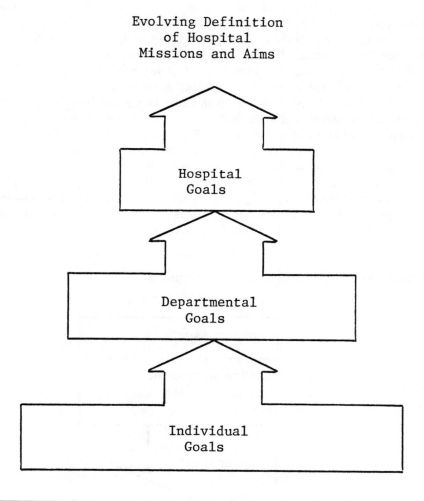

Evolving Definition
of Hospital
Missions and Aims

Hospital
Goals

Departmental
Goals

Individual
Goals

promote overall organizational performance. Obviously, for example, the medical records department cannot process records (and claims) if nursing units are delaying completion of the records after patient discharge. The medical records department should not be penalized for events beyond its control, but the nursing department may be penalized for creating this sort of obstruction.

## SETTING STANDARDS FOR PERFORMANCE

The advent of DRG-based prospective payment will require hospitals to upgrade their standards of performance to ensure better attainment of financial goals. At the department level, the department heads and supervisors can and should take responsibility for the improvement in standards. Therefore, prospective payment will modify the very association between supervisor and individual staff members (Figure 13–3). This fact presents no unusual dilemmas as long as supervisors recognize that they must change their own patterns of behavior while helping staff members improve their individual capabilities.

The first responsibility of supervisors in setting higher standards for performance is to help subordinates define performance criteria. Head nurses must move beyond abstract terms of efficiency and effectiveness to specific definitions of better nursing performance. The purchasing manager must work with an inventory clerk in defining new standards of personal productivity and methods by which those standards can be attained. Food service managers must help kitchen aides understand how their productivity must improve; what that higher productivity means precisely in terms of meals served, dishes washed, or patients satisfied; and how they might begin to achieve this better performance.

---

**Figure 13–3** Setting Standards for Performance

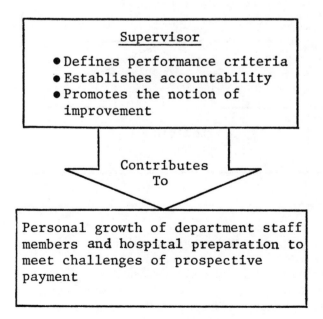

Supervisors will also be expected to establish accountability under prospective payment. Because hospitals need to contain costs, to increase productivity, and to improve quality under DRG-based reimbursement, they will not be able to subsidize poor employee performance. Department heads will play a particularly critical role in establishing and reinforcing employees' accountability.

Finally, supervisors must promote the notion of improvement. There is always a higher performance standard toward which humans can strive. This is the time for surgeons who are operating, for accountants who are reviewing cost records, for nurses who are caring for patients, and for medical technicians who are drawing blood to strive for their best. Many staff members are too easily swayed to complacency. The daily give and take of work may desensitize employees to their lack of progress toward high goals. With the assistance of the department head and the supervisor, however, hospital employees can move from a mundane and routine performance to one that contributes to the hospital's battle with cost control.

---

**NOTES**

1. Gary P. Latham and James J. Baldes, "The 'Practical Significance' of Locke's Theory of Goal Setting," *Journal of Applied Psychology* 60 (1975): 122–124.

2. Gary P. Latham and Gary A. Yukl, "Effects of Assigned and Participative Goal Setting on Performance and Job Satisfaction," *Journal of Applied Psychology* 61 (1976): 166–171.

3. John N. Ivancevich, "Effects of Goal Setting on Performance and Job Satisfaction," *Journal of Applied Psychology* 61 (1976): 605–612.

4. Jay S. Kim and W. Clay Hammer, "Effect of Performance Feedback and Goal Setting on Productivity and Satisfaction in an Organizational Setting," *Journal of Applied Psychology* 61 (1976): 48–57.

5. John N. Ivancevich, "Different Goal Setting Treatments and Their Effects on Performance and Job Satisfaction," *Academy of Management Journal* 20 (1977): 406–419.

6. William J. Kearney, "Improving Work Performance through Appraisal," *Human Resource Management* 13 (1978): 15–23.

7. Douglas McGregor, "An Uneasy Look at Performance Appraisal," *Harvard Business Review* 59 (1972): 133–138.

# Chapter 14

# The Future of Prospective Payment Systems

There is no crystal ball that can accurately predict what the future holds for hospitals and other health care institutions under prospective payment systems. It is safe to say, however, that a prospective payment system of some sort is here to stay. This radical change in the way hospitals are reimbursed for their services is the most important change in our health care delivery system since the introduction of Medicare and Medicaid in the mid-1960s.

Obviously, the future of the prospective payment system for Medicare rests with the U.S. Congress. It has yet to be determined whether Medicare will continue to use diagnosis-related groups (DRGs) as a basis for reimbursement, but the most likely scenario is continual modification and refinement of the present system, together with extension of the prospective payment system to other third party payers. Hospitals should assume that prospective reimbursement is here to stay and make every effort to adapt to this change.

It is difficult to predict specific congressional action on prospective reimbursement because, until the system has been operating for three or four years on a national level, it will not be known whether it provides a sound basis for a national system of prospective budgeting.[1] Nevertheless, the broad outlines of the future are now readily discernible in the current social trends that are not easily reversed (Figure 14–1).

Changes in the external environment will force hospitals to make managerial changes. Costs will continue to rise, although at a somewhat slower rate. The enormous and increasing amount of resources being devoted to health care will generate philosophical and attitudinal changes in the American people and their representatives. These changes, in turn, are expected to increase *both* government regulation and competition, as well as to slow the rate of growth in health care resources. Obviously, these trends will create special problems and opportunities for hospitals that can be addressed by developing new strategies and operational procedures that may eventually moderate the rate of increase in costs.

231

**Figure 14–1** A Conceptual Framework for Forecasting Future Changes in the U.S. Health Care System and Their Impact on Hospital Management

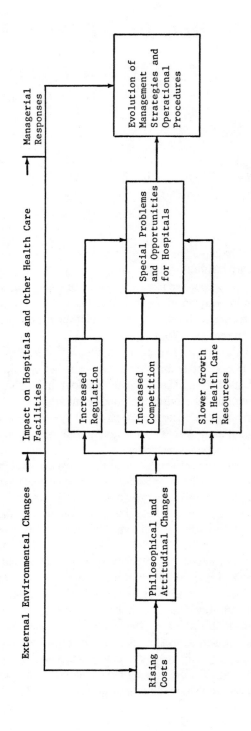

## PHILOSOPHICAL AND ATTITUDINAL CHANGES

Most Americans have made some contribution to the problem of rising health care costs, and there is no evidence that we are willing to accept changes that would adversely affect our own interests in the short run.[2] The coming physician surplus is likely to contribute to the cost spiral, since it will probably increase the use of medical services. After years of sacrifice, physicians feel entitled to a high salary, as do the growing numbers of allied health professionals. Private companies operating in the industry also feel entitled to a good profit. The middle class now expects medical insurance to pay for most medical care expenses instead of only those associated with catastrophic illness and accident. Finally, the "baby boom" generation is coming of age and demanding more medical care services just as technological advances have expanded the possibilities for prolonging human life.

Congress continues to increase federal appropriations for favored groups in the population. Between 1968 and 1980, for example, medical payments for veterans jumped 410 percent, from $1.6 billion to $6.6 billion.[3] This rate of increase has continued under the Reagan Administration. Between 1960 and 1980, the number of recipients of Aid to Families with Dependent Children jumped from 3 million to 11 million, and all these individuals entered the Medicaid program.

The inevitable conclusion is that health care costs are uncontrollable in the short run and can be controlled in the long run only if we are willing to deny medical services to certain individuals under certain circumstances. At present, however, we have no way to make such judgments. We want lower costs, but we want medical treatment available to everyone. The burgeoning costs of health care will undoubtedly result in some changes in societal values, as well as some form of rationing for medical services. The most important philosophical ideas that may undergo change include the following:[4]

- *Health care is a right.* This concept is consistent with the egalitarian, democratic belief that everyone should have equal access to health services and the best medical technology available. Yet, those dependent on Medicare or Medicaid are already at a disadvantage compared with those covered by private insurance. This gap will continue to widen in the years ahead as the tax burden increases.

- *The hospital is a service, not a business.* More hospitals are being run as businesses today, and this trend will increase in the future because of the economic pressures.

- *Good health requires high technology medical care.* There may be a shift from high-technology to low-technology medical care.

- *The hospital is the hub of health care.* Health care is now being decentralized and deinstitutionalized. Americans are moving away from institutionalized medicine by taking more responsibility for their own health.[5]

## INCREASED REGULATION AND COMPETITION

The impact of our changing philosophies and attitudes may well be a paradoxical combination of more regulation and more competition. While the two are generally considered alternatives, they may well be complementary approaches to cost containment.

### Regulatory Changes and Impacts

Regulatory bodies are here to stay in health care, whether they take the form of government rate commissions or government-controlled health care systems. Formats or allocation of authority may change, but some form of regulatory control will exist for many years in the future.

#### Rationing

Effective control of spiraling U.S. health care costs will require some form of rationing. Some services will have to be withheld from at least some patients, as they have been in Great Britain.[6] In fact, many of the patterns evident in Great Britain will appear in the United States when the cost problem reaches a crisis and forces an effective cost containment program. U.S. physicians will have to weigh the relative costs and benefits of different forms of care for particular patients. They will also have to decide what care not to provide, based on the age of the patient. This will mean care that is dependent on costly capital equipment will be constrained, since such decisions concerning how much to invest can be made impersonally. The availability and use of such technology will be more heavily regulated in order to relieve physicians of difficult moral choices.

#### Restrictions on New Technology

Health care has always been technology-driven, and dramatic advances in technology have changed patient care over the years. Now that hospitals must provide a service on a price-specific basis, they must assess products on the basis of *both* clinical outcome and cost.[7] The question is not what will cost least by itself, but what will cost least in the overall treatment of the patient from admission to discharge. Because of this growing suspicion that the additional social benefits do not justify the social costs, the introduction of new technology and services is likely to be a controversial issue over the next decade. Regulators face the difficult task of developing methods by which to separate cost-effective equipment and services from those that are cost-ineffective.[8]

The Office of Technology Assessment has concluded that hospitals will buy less cost-increasing capital equipment under prospective reimbursement.[9] It also raised the question of how the new reimbursement system will affect technological change in medicine, the adoption of new technologies, and the rejection of old ones, noting that some patients may be denied access to significant medical advances. The Department of Health and Human Services submitted a report to Congress in October 1984 on the various ways to incorporate capital costs into the DRG system. Implementation of capital cost prospective payment could have negative implications for the growth of medical technology.

### Hospital Survival

Prospective reimbursement is likely to result in revenue cuts that will make it increasingly difficult for hospitals to attract the capital necessary for survival. Capacity reductions should follow shortly. It is very likely that there will be fewer hospitals, fewer hospital beds, and fewer patient days under the new system.[10,11] Therefore, hospitals will be competing for patient days, and some will go out of business. Some observers predict that as many as 1,000 hospitals will close in the next decade.

Many feel that the new system will accelerate the shift away from free-standing hospitals, give hospital systems the opportunity to acquire smaller hospitals, and generally benefit the hospital chains, which are considered more efficient and better able to generate capital internally.[12] The accelerated demise of small free-standing hospitals will be due to the cost of management systems necessary to comply with prospective payment requirements. Most free-standing hospitals will be acquired by investor-owned and nonprofit multihospital systems. However, a consolidated system with fewer hospitals can expect more government pressure to regulate their behavior and to apply rigorous antitrust action.[13]

While many are concerned that the new reimbursement system will adversely affect the quality of patient care,[14] others are more sanguine.[15] Prospective payment imposes constraints on the rate at which quality can improve by placing limits on revenue, but quality need not deteriorate below existing levels so long as the payment rates cover current services furnished in an efficient manner.[16] Efforts to function efficiently are not necessarily inconsistent with the goal of providing top-notch care. Quality may even improve if hospitals with a low patient volume cease to render services that can be provided efficiently and effectively only when volume is high.[17]

### Modification and Extension of Prospective Payment Systems

The prospective pricing system can be expected to survive (in some form) and to spread to other third party payers. If the Medicare DRG-based system proves effective, other third party payers will follow suit very quickly. Most state Medicaid directors now expect that their programs will build a new prospective reimbursement system modeled along the lines of the federal Medicare system.[18] Furthermore, Medicare prospective rates will eventually be made available for use by other third party insurers. Lest hospitals think that prospective payment will be limited to patient care, the Health Care Financing Administration (HCFA) plans to extend the concept to skilled nursing and outpatient care, as well as to care provided by physicians.[19]

The inclusion of physicians will be a major modification of the existing Medicare system, but the present dichotomy in which the hospital care provided to Medicare patients is divided into institutional and professional components with opposing incentives cannot persist indefinitely. First, it conflicts with the notion of paying flat amounts for specific illnesses, since the payment actually covers only a portion of the services provided. Second, Medicare spending may not be effectively curtailed if charges can be shifted from the hospital to the physician. Third, the law instructs the secretary of Health and Human Services to collect data needed to compute DRG-specific physician charges and to report to Congress in 1985 about the advisability and feasibility of paying physicians on a prospective basis.[20] In December 1984, the Reagan Administration proposed a freeze on physician payments for Medicare patients.

One other possible change that would affect physicians is the adoption of a "mandatory assignment" provision or regulation.[21] Such a provision would require physicians to accept the Medicare payment as the full payment for services and prohibit them from billing Medicare recipients for an extra charge. Assignment is voluntary now. Congressional proposals have linked mandatory assignment to a freeze on physician fees. Supporters argue that physicians might refuse to take assignment so that they could bill Medicare beneficiaries directly to compensate for the frozen Medicare payments. Opponents have argued that enactment of these proposals would hurt Medicare recipients because many physicians may stop treating Medicare beneficiaries if assignment is mandated; they prefer to create incentives, such as priority claims handling, to encourage physicians to take assignment.

The integration of physician payment into the DRG-based reimbursement system also raises other questions:[22]

- Should the hospital receive payment and then pay the physician or vice versa?
- Should the physician who hospitalized the patient receive payment and then pay other physicians?

These issues are presently being studied by the HCFA. In addition, the HCFA is studying the advisability of incorporating alternate delivery systems, such as health maintenance organizations, into the Medicare system; a voucher system; caps on tax-free insurance benefits; and more cost sharing by Medicaid beneficiaries.

Much refining will be necessary before the Medicare prospective payment system reaches its potential. Examination of various case mix methods, such as patient management categories that stress optimal (as opposed to average) patient management, and modification of the existing system to consider severity of illness are clearly in order.

In the meantime, many states are taking action to reduce their expenditure for Medicaid, sometimes with dramatic results.[23] Among the methods being used are restrictions on the use of inpatient hospital services, co-payments, reduced availability of services, tighter eligibility requirements, implementation of prospective payment systems, prior authorization for various services, and strategies to control fraud and abuse.

## Competitive Changes and Impacts

Advocates of the competitive approach to hospital reimbursement believe that the removal of various restraints to competition in health care will encourage innovation and cost containment as it has in other industries. They believe that the consumer, by making rational choices regarding health care services, can contain the rate of increase in health care costs.[24] Indeed, recent research indicates that one approach to competition, cost sharing by consumers, results in lower health care expenditures.[25]

The competitive approach could be put into practice as a voucher system. Annually, each U.S. family would receive a voucher worth a fixed amount of money from the federal government; the voucher could be used only to purchase health care services. Free to supplement this with their own resources, consumers would select from among several providers, based on perceptions of quality and price. The idea is to focus on total (rather than unit) health care expenditures and to create incentives for providers to compete for the consumers' health care dollar. Altman has predicted a move to a voucher system, possibly by the late 1980s,[26] but he has also cautioned that more research is needed to determine the amount appropriate for the vouchers.

Information about DRG-specific costs for Medicare and non-Medicare patients may also encourage more competition among hospitals.[27] Hospitals with low occupancy rates, for example, may use DRG cost information to bid for contracts with other hospitals, health maintenance organizations, employers, employer coalitions, or other organizations. In this way, they could become preferred provider organizations for some or all DRGs.

Similarly, Medicare itself may someday attempt to enhance competition through the use of vouchers and beneficiaries. The program may also require hospitals to bid for Medicare patients.[28] California is already using this approach for Medicaid patients. Medicare may award contracts for hospital care to the lowest bidders and pay the awarded rates to all hospitals. Medicare recipients who elect treatment in more expensive hospitals may be required to pay the cost differential. This approach may well reduce such cost differentials over time. In such a competitive environment, hospitals with cost-effective medical technology and no teaching costs may have a cost advantage over other hospitals.

Other manifestations of an increasingly competitive environment are recent court decisions regarding the role of various medical associations.[29] Since the Supreme Court ruled in the mid-1970s that the "learned professions" are subject to antitrust laws, the American Medical Association has been sued for its ban on advertising; lower courts have upheld a Federal Trade Commission ruling that such restraint is anticompetitive. Other medical association regulations that have been ruled anticompetitive include a fee schedule set by the county medical society, refusal to reimburse nonphysicians, physician-controlled prepaid medical insurance, and boycotts of health maintenance organizations.

As a consequence of these legal precedents, as well as the growing oversupply of U.S. physicians, there will be several developments over the next decade. Physician-controlled emergency centers will pull profits away from hospital laboratory, surgery, and radiology services.[30] Medical treatments for such conditions as obesity, behavioral problems, and sports injuries will increase.[31] More care may be provided to "less desirable" patients, such as those in prisons, mental institutions, and long-term care facilities, as well as to the chronically ill and the elderly confined to their homes. Physicians may also provide more convenient office hours, walk-in services, and free consultations.

As a result of all these changes, there may be fierce competition and territorial battles between physicians and hospitals, hospitals and hospitals, hospitals and ambulatory facilities, physicians and physicians, and physicians and nurses.[32] The increased competition throughout the health care industry may be expected to create downward pressure on costs. The environmental changes may also slow improvements in access and quality, however, while threatening the existence or local control of some hospitals. It remains to be seen whether the public will accept these changes.

## FUTURE STRATEGIES AND OPERATIONAL APPROACHES

According to Naisbett and Elkins, hospitals will have to reconceptualize their business to fit into the wellness trend.[33] This requires a dramatic change in role for most hospitals, since they must shift their focus from short-term treatment of illness to long-term support of wellness. For most institutions, such a radical change can be made only over the long run. In the meantime, there are several less radical strategies and procedures that should be implemented over the next five years to help a hospital survive.

## Data Collection and Analysis

Hospitals must immediately implement a management information system that can provide their net profit by DRG and by physician. Such data will allow them to identify those DRGs that they can treat profitably and to decide whether to specialize in those cases. Specialization within hospitals is expected to increase as management focuses on those DRGs for which the institution has some competitive advantage. Those hospitals with the necessary information system in place will be at a distinct advantage in determining which DRGs are profitable to them and which are eroding their financial viability.

Hospitals will probably find the treatment of routine cases more profitable than the treatment of complex cases under a fixed payment rate based on average costs.[34] Some of the costs of complicated cases have traditionally been allocated to routine cases; now that this is no longer done, less complicated DRGs have more attractive payment rates. As a result, hospitals will compete for certain types of lucrative cases and will shun less profitable cases. Patients may have to wait to gain admission to a hospital for treatment of less profitable ailments. At some point, the reimbursement rate differentials will probably be adjusted by the HCFA.

Some experts believe that hospitals will drop those inpatient services that do not provide them with a respectable profit. Others believe that, while hospitals may change their service mix to attract more patients who fall into financially attractive DRGs, they will continue to provide all services in order to attract as many patients as possible.[35] Furthermore, Medicare will pay more than it costs to provide treatment for particular DRGs. Less than half of the DRG rate will be tied directly to the costs of providing care. The rest will be based on the fixed costs that the hospital must pay anyway. Therefore, the true cost of treating a particular patient is not the average cost, but the incremental or variable cost associated with that care (i.e., food and drugs).

Researchers contend that as much as 60 percent of a hospital's costs may be fixed costs.[36] About 60 percent of all DRG payments comes from costs incurred in treating all patients (fixed costs), rather than any particular patient (variable costs). Thus, the cost of treating each Medicare patient is only 40 percent of the DRG payment. A hospital gearing up for the DRG system should not measure "profit" and "loss" per DRG on the basis of average cost, but on the basis of what Medicare pays for each DRG and its variable cost for each DRG. The difference represents the key number—the contribution margin for each DRG.

## Strategic Planning

In order to survive over the next decade, hospitals will need to develop a strategic plan. Because it is likely that hospitals will be asked to be the allocators of health care resources in the future, at least in part,[37] it will be increasingly important to have a consensus among the institutional leaders about the mission and future direction of the hospital. Such a consensus can be developed if there is a clear understanding that implementation of the necessary changes may make funds available to implement additional objectives in the strategic plan.

The new reimbursement system provides incentives for hospitals to become vertically and horizontally integrated. As long as Medicare faces a huge deficit, it will be pressured by Congress to favor aftercare over acute care, and hospitals will have an incentive to become vertically integrated by buying nursing homes and other chronic care facilities. The shift in emphasis from the short-term treatment of illness to the long-term support of wellness will reinforce this trend.[38]

There is an incentive under prospective reimbursement to perform diagnostic work *before* patients are admitted to the hospital and to use the hospital strictly for patient treatment.[39] There are virtually no restrictions on reimbursement for care provided outside the hospital. Some hospitals have responded to this circumstance by establishing free-standing diagnostic imaging centers as a form of vertical integration.

Both investor-owned and nonprofit hospitals will become more horizontally integrated as they buy for-profit businesses in order to raise capital. Since financial rating agencies like Moodys have already begun to downgrade hospital ratings as a result of prospective reimbursement, hospitals will experience increased difficulty in raising money and will pay more for it. Vertical expansion into profitable health and non–health-related businesses is the logical outcome of this constraint.

Some hospitals are forming joint ventures with their medical staffs to share risk and responsibility for performance under prospective payment systems, Medicaid competitive contracting programs, and private alternate delivery systems.[40] Together, they organize the participating physicians, negotiate risk-sharing contracts with payers, operate the utilization control and quality assurance systems, and distribute the profit or losses.

## Management of Change

The new reimbursement system necessitates a supportive organizational climate.[41] An extensive communications effort must be aimed at changing goals, attitudes, and behavior. In particular, the trustees and the medical staff must understand the causes of hospital cost increases, the way in which prospective reimbursement is designed to deal with the problem, and the implications of prospective reimbursement for the hospital.

There also must be more physician involvement in hospital management.[42] In the future, physicians will be more involved in planning, delivering, monitoring, and controlling functions. In some hospitals, physicians already occupy positions in marketing and operations, and more are serving as chief executive officers. Since product lines must be defined for payment purposes and the definitions of product lines are clinically based, physicians may well become hospital product line managers as well. Management must produce clinical and cost information on a patient-specific basis so those physicians within a clinical specialty will be able to review and monitor their treatment of patients.

Since physicians are the major decision makers regarding the utilization of hospital resources, they should be actively involved in any program that controls admissions, length of stay, and ancillary service usage.[43] Physicians should be analyzing clinical and financial data on resource use and providing clinical input to the hospital's resource allocation decision process. Administrators should involve physicians in any and all decisions relating to the inputs required to treat patients. It may be necessary to create or expand formal structures that involve physicians in controlling resource use.

The decisions facing hospitals will require the cooperation of many different professionals in the organization. The DRG task force or committee is a useful mechanism for allowing inputs from nonphysician staff members. The committee should have real authority if it is to be viewed as anything other than "window dressing," however.

### Productivity Management

While hospitals will continue to manage the functional aspects of services, such as nursing and laboratory services, they will need to identify specific product lines and product line managers. These individuals will be responsible for productivity, monitoring and control, advertising and marketing, and quality assurance.[44] Improvements in productivity are more likely when a specific individual is held responsible for specific results.

The product line manager or department head must identify problem areas, propose improvements, and gain employee acceptance of whatever changes seem appropriate. Once opportunities for increasing productivity have been identified, an effective management engineering program will be needed to permit further analysis, development, implementation, and evaluation of needed changes in hospital operations. Behavioral science approaches may be applied to increase employee motivation for productivity improvement. The rate of increase in employee productivity will also be dependent on how well department or product line managers control resource use (i.e., inputs). This necessitates a patient-based information system that allows comparisons of resource use patterns among groups of similar patients.[45]

## CONCLUSION

At this point, it is unclear whether DRG-based reimbursement will really effect fundamental reform or whether it will just create a new reimbursement "game." For example, highly variable costs within a DRG could cause hospitals to juggle the reimbursement system to maximize their payments.[46] In such a case, Congress might well abandon the prospective payment approach and adopt a more rigid regulatory apparatus under some type of national health insurance program. Over the next five years, however, the prospective payment system will probably be tested, modified, and extended. As such, it may well constitute the last opportunity that hospitals will have to reform their own management systems voluntarily in order to improve both quality and efficiency.

---

**NOTES**

1. Eli Ginzberg, "Cost Containment—Imaginary and Real," *New England Journal of Medicine* 308 (May 1983): 1220–1224.

2. Gregory E. Pence, "Everyone's Entitled To Blame for Soaring Health Costs," *Wall Street Journal,* December 22, 1983, 24.

3. Ibid.

4. Eleanor S. Schrader, "Will DRGs Change Our Ideas about What Health Care Means?" *AORN Journal* 38 (November 1983): 752–754.

5. John Naisbett and John Elkins, "The Hospital and Megatrends," *Hospital Forum* 26 (July-August 1983): 54.

6. Henry J. Aaron and William B. Schwartz, *The Painful Prescription: Rationing Health Care* (Washington, D.C.: The Brookings Institution, 1984).

7. John G. Nackel, P. Douglas Powell, and Michael J. Goran, "Case Mix Management: Issues and Strategies," *Hospital and Health Services Administration* 29 (January-February 1984): 9–10.

8. Paul L. Grimaldi, "Prospective Payment Scheme Overhauls Hospitals' Financial Incentives," *Hospital Progress* 65 (August 1983): 50.

9. U.S. Department of Health and Human Services, Office of Technology Assessment, *Diagnosis-Related Groups and the Medicine Program: Implications for Medical Technology* (Washington, D.C.: U.S. Government Printing Office, 1983).

10. Nackel, Powell, and Goran, "Case Mix Management," 11.

11. Montague Brown, "From the Editor," *Health Care Management Review* 8 (Summer 1983): 5–6.

12. "Analysts Predict Good Future for Hospital Stocks," *Hospitals* 57 (December 1, 1983): 42.

13. Brown, "From the Editor."

14. Lynn Kahn, "Meeting of the Minds: Hospital/Physician Diplomacy Crucial under Prospective System," *Hospitals* 57 (March 16, 1983): 84–86.

15. Grimaldi, "Prospective Payment Scheme Overhauls Hospitals' Financial Incentives."

16. Ibid.

17. Ann Barry Flood, W. Richard Scott, and Wayne Ewy, "Does Practice Make Perfect? The Relationship between Hospital Volume and Outcomes for Selected Diagnostic Categories," *Medical Care* 22 (February 1984): 98–114.

18. "Medicare May Have Domino Effect on Medicaid Plans," *Modern Healthcare* 13 (September 1983): 54.

19. "Speaker Relates New Jersey Hospitals' DRG Experiences." *Hospitals* 57 (April 16, 1983): 38.

20. Grimaldi, "Prospective Payment Scheme Overhauls Hospitals' Financial Incentives."

21. Cynthia Wallace, "Congress Already Debating Prospective Pay Changes," *Modern Healthcare* 13 (December 1983): 22.

22. "For-Profits' Meeting Examines DRG System, Capital Payment Options," *Hospital Progress* 66 (April 1984): 20–21.

23. "States Rein in Costs, Get Dramatic Results," *Modern Healthcare* 13 (March 1983): 74.

24. Alan A. Enthoven, "The Competition Strategy: Status and Prospects," *New England Journal of Medicine* 304 (January 1981): 109–112.

25. Joseph P. Newhouse, "Some Interim Results from a Controlled Trial of Cost Sharing in Health Insurance," *New England Journal of Medicine* 305 (December 1981): 1501–1507.

26. "For-Profits' Meeting Examines DRG System, Capital Payment Options."

27. Grimaldi, "Prospective Payment Scheme Overhauls Hospitals' Financial Incentives."

28. Ibid.

29. "The Spiraling Costs of Health Care," *Business Week,* February 8, 1982, 61.

30. Paul Ellwood and Linda Ellwein, "Physician Glut Will Force Hospitals To Look Outward," *Hospitals* 55 (January 15, 1981): 81.

31. Emily Friedman, "Doctor, the Patient Will See You Now," *Hospitals* 55 (September 16, 1981): 117.

32. Donna Richards Sheridan, "The Health Care Industry in the Marketplace: Implications for Nursing," *The Journal of Nursing Administration* 13 (September 1983): 38.

33. Naisbett and Elkins, "The Hospital and Megatrends," 55.

34. "Prospective Pricing Expected to Raise Hospitals' Financial Risk," *Hospitals* 57 (April 16, 1983): 23.

35. Arthur J. Keegan, "Hospitals Will Continue To Treat All DRGs To Snare Contribution Margin," *Modern Healthcare* 13 (September 1983): 206.

36. Ibid.

37. William R. Fifer, "Cost/Quality Tradeoffs Will Be the Next Medical Care Crisis," *Hospitals* 55 (June 1981): 56–59.

38. Naisbett and Elkins, "The Hospital and Megatrends."

39. "PPS's Push for Outpatient Diagnostic Work Is the Catalyst," *Hospitals* 57 (November 16, 1983): 44.

40. Nackel, Powell, and Goran, "Case Mix Management," 13.

41. M. Orry Jacobs, "Competition and Regulation: Do They Make a Difference in Hospital Reimbursement? " *Health Care Management Review* 8 (Summer 1983): 53–56.

42. Nackel, Powell, and Goran, "Case Mix Management," 8.

43. Jacobs, "Competition and Regulation," 56.

44. Nackel, Powell, and Goran, "Case Mix Management," 12.

45. Jacobs, "Competition and Regulation," 56.

46. Marlene Bloom, "Enthoven Calls DRG Plan Temporary," *Hospitals* 57 (February 1, 1983): 20.

# Index

---

*Note:* Page numbers in *italics* indicate entry will be found in figures or tables.

# O

# P

# About the Authors

**Howard L. Smith, Ph.D.,** received his masters degree in health planning from UCLA and his doctorate in administrative theory from the University of Washington. Currently, he is an Associate Professor in the Department of Health Administration at the Medical College of Virginia in Richmond, Virginia where he teaches health care finance, strategic planning and marketing, and long-term care administration. Dr. Smith has published and consulted extensively in the health services administration field, particularly in the areas of strategic management, planning, physician management, and cost containment. Recently, he served as a consultant to several developing countries on improving operations in their primary health care systems.

**Myron D. Fottler, Ph.D.,** is currently Professor of Management and Director of the Ph.D. Program in Administration-Health Services with a joint appointment in the Graduate School of Management and the School of Community and Allied Health, University of Alabama at Birmingham. In addition to teaching courses in human resources management, he has more than 100 publications in the areas of health care cost containment, human resources problems in health care, human resources development, multi-institutional systems, and other areas of health care administration and policy. He is the 1985 Chairperson of the Health Care Administration Division of the Academy of Management. His biography has been listed in several publications including *Who's Who in the East, Contemporary Authors, Outstanding Young Men in America, Dictionary of International Biography, International Writers and Authors Who's Who,* and *American Men and Women of Science.*